Letters from Liberia

The Adventures of an Ebola Medical Volunteer

Joe Spann, M.D.

DEDICATED TO THE PEOPLE OF
LIBERIA AND THE MEDICAL WORKERS
INVOLVED IN THE EBOLA EPIDEMIC
OF 2014-2015

ISBN: 1508735786
ISBN-13: 9781508735786

Contents

PREFACE

This book is a compilation of letters and stories that I wrote to my family and friends during the time I was in Liberia as an Ebola medical volunteer. The letters were meant to be informative on what I was seeing and doing in Liberia but ended up being much more. The overall experience was not what I had expected, filled with more joy and surprises than sadness and death. I think the take home message is to never be afraid to follow your faith and heart when you are called to action on behalf of others.

I would like to thank the American Refugee Committee for allowing me to be a part of their Liberia Ebola Emergency Response Team.

Thanks to Russell Secker for his expertise in the publishing process of this book.

Thanks also to Amy Sharp for her expert editing and advice and to my neighbor, Jack London, for his astute writing tips and encouragement.

Special gratitude and love to my wife, June, who provided additional editing and advice and tolerated my long absence from home.

Lastly, my greatest praise to those individuals who lived and worked with me while deployed in Liberia especially Jonathan, Kelsy, Mark, Cher, Isaac, John, Demenia, Doris, George and Henry. Without you, none of this would have ever happened.

Dr. Joe Spann

Suiting Up for Battle

I had been watching the news and thinking about Ebola for several weeks. The Ebola epidemic had taken thousands of lives in West Africa, and the World Health Organization was predicting over 100,000 deaths in the next few months if the Ebola epidemic was not brought under control. At the same time several healthcare workers had been brought back to the United States deathly ill as a result of working with Ebola patients.

As many others did, I thought, "Someone should go stop this virus before it spreads to the United States and kills us all!" I was also thinking, "Someone should go help those poor people in West Africa!"

Having spent the first half of my adult life following the self-centered principles outlined by popular rock and roll lyrics, I decided that I should try some alternative ideas, so I joined a Bible study group at my local church. We were studying the book of Ephesians, which is most well-known for a call to action against the evils of the world:

"We are not fighting against flesh-and-blood enemies, but against evil rulers and authorities of the unseen world, against mighty powers in this dark world, and against evil spirits in the heavenly places." Ephesians 6:12.

Being a medical doctor and therefore a scientist by training, I dissected this phrase and examined it closely: "Not flesh and blood", "unseen world", and "dark world." I interpreted this as a microscopic enemy hidden in a dark continent: Ebola in Africa.

In the next section of Ephesians we are told to suit up for battle in all of God's armor:

" Wear the belt of truth, and put on the breastplate of righteousness, shoes to proclaim the gospel of peace, the helmet of salvation and take the shield of faith to quench all the flaming arrows of the evil one." Ephesians 6:13-17.

I envisioned the photos I had seen on TV and in newspapers of the Ebola workers in Africa wearing their protective gear used in Ebola treatment areas: the suits, the aprons, the boots, the hoods, and the masks. Could this not be God's armor? Or had I stumbled across the worse allegory ever?

So I pondered the coincidences, implications, and meaning of this in my life. I was a relatively young, retired physician trained in general medicine. My children were grown and independent, both of my parents were deceased, and my wife was healthy and financially secure. The only creature remotely dependent upon me was the dog, and I was pretty sure she could get by without me.

Unlike other battles in our world, the fight against Ebola would not require a military army, but an army of healthcare workers. This time the "someone" who should go fight Ebola and help the people of West Africa was in the mirror, staring back at me. And so, I decided to suit up for battle against Ebola.

After a quick Internet search I was in contact with the American Refugee Committee (ARC) based in Minneapolis, Minnesota. I had never heard of them before, but a friend recommended them, and ARC received favorable comments on the Internet. I sent in my CV and references, underwent a telephone interview, and waited.

The next week I was accepted to work as a medical doctor on the Ebola Emergency Response Team sponsored by ARC. I was tempted to ask how many physicians applied for my position but was afraid to know the answer. We would be based in Fish Town, Liberia for approximately 3 months to work in a soon to be constructed Ebola Treatment Unit (ETU). I liked the sound of Fish Town as my deployment base, and I took this as a good sign. The bigger question was should I pack a fishing rod?

Our medical team would meet for the first time in Minneapolis in mid-November at ARC headquarters. We would have several days of orientation and then ship out to Liberia. I didn't know any of the nurses or doctors that would be with me for the next 3 months. It was time to make some new friends.

I spoke with and sent e-mails to all of my family informing them of my decision to go to Liberia to fight Ebola. I received the most loving and supportive responses you could ever imagine. A few tried to talk me out of it, but knew I was too stubborn to change my mind.

My wife, June, and I celebrated our 34th wedding anniversary on November 15th, 2014. After that it was time to gather up the full armor of God and fly to Minneapolis. I just hope I have enough room in my suitcase for all the extra weight and space required for the armor.

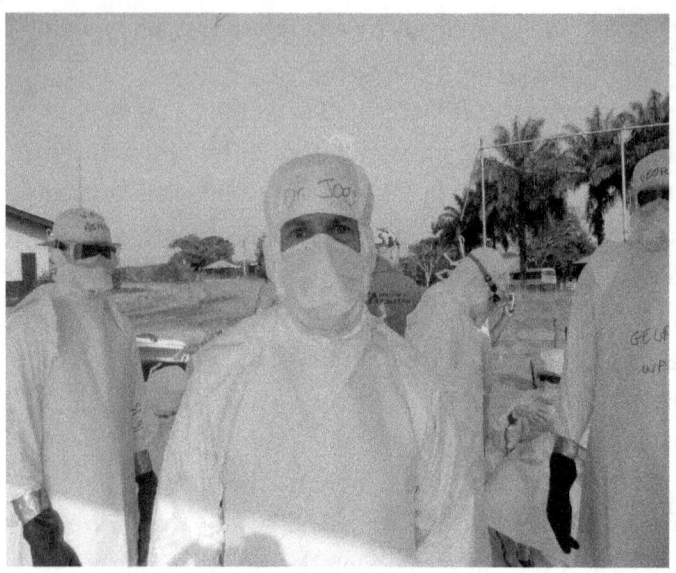

Dr. Joe in his armor.

Letter to My Family

Wednesday, October 29, 2014

Dear Family,

I think everyone is aware of the medical and humanitarian crisis that has been going on in West Africa the past few months. The Ebola virus is a nasty bug, but it has been particularly deadly in a region of the world already devastated by poverty, civil war, and lack of an adequate medical infrastructure. However, with basic medical care it can be treated, survived, and eventually eliminated.

We are entering a period of time now where maximal medical resources and personnel need to be utilized to contain this deadly disease. If it should spread to other densely populated and impoverished countries, such as India or China, there could be catastrophic loss of life.

I have volunteered to work with the American Refugee Committee (ARC) that is based in Minneapolis, Minnesota. It is a reputable non-profit group that provides assistance to refugees and disadvantaged persons around the world. I will be working with qualified doctors, nurses, and other health care personnel.

My tour will begin on November 17th and will last for approximately 3 months. I will be flown to Minnesota initially to meet my team (8 – 12 volunteers) and begin training. We will then leave from there to Monrovia, Liberia on Nov. 20th. I will spend 7 days in Bong County being trained in the Ebola Treatment Unit (ETU) operated by the International Medical Corp. Afterwards, I will travel by 4-wheel drive truck or SUV to Fish Town, Liberia. (Yes, I am bringing my fishing pole!)

Our team will be the first to utilize the newly built ETU and will have newly built housing in which to sleep and live. There will be Internet access, and I hope to keep in touch with all of you so I don't go completely mad. I hope to learn to Skype successfully and will utilize that as much as possible.   I will try to send out periodic updates on what is going on in my life, and I hope to keep up with yours.

ARC is going to provide the best training, medical supplies, and technical support that are currently available. I believe that the protective gowns and sanitation protocols are going to work successfully. If not, I get a free ride out of Liberia to a stateside Ebola treatment hospital of my choice.

I am sorry I will miss the 2014 holidays with you, but I promise to return to aggravate everyone a few more times. I tentatively plan to return to the United States in mid-February 2015.

I'm not sure where my 21- day quarantine will take place. I 'm hoping for Las Vegas.

Love,

Joe

Taking Off

November 17th, 2014

Dear Family and Friends,

It has been a busy weekend with packing, my wedding anniversary, repacking, farewell dinners with family and friends, re-repacking, etc. There was an article in the local newspaper about my upcoming trip to Liberia to fight Ebola. I received many supportive and kind phone calls, e-mails, and letters. There was even an announcement at our church where many members sympathetically looked upon me as one headed towards certain doom. Wrong! Armor of God folks!

It was a relief to finally be heading out to the airport Monday afternoon. The final summation of my gear was two suitcases weighing 50 pounds apiece and a carry-on backpack weighing 25 pounds. I packed items that are silly and unnecessary but were given to me by friends and relatives for love, good luck, or possible use that I must take with me.

I have a small Bible that was carried by my father-in-law during WWII and a commemorative silver coin from the Marines' Memorial Association given to me by my dear cousin Dianne and her gentleman ex-Marine husband, Jon. I have a small photo book filled with pictures of family and friends. There is also a Snake Farm coffee cup along with a Wally World glass moose mug given to me by my daughter, Ellen. Lastly, I have a rubber snake presented to me by my good friend Steve for security purposes. He has spent time in Africa before and assures me a rubber snake is the ultimate protection against thievery.

I received a loving farewell from my super wife, June, and flew to Houston just in time for a flight delay to Minneapolis. Fortunately, I had a United Club pass, and I was able to drink 2 free beers in relative solitude while awaiting my next flight.

At 5 p.m. the direct flight to Minneapolis took off, and we arrived a little after 8 p.m. My taxi driver spoke little English and had to use a smartphone to lookup the location of my downtown hotel, a Holiday Inn Express. I was finally able to check-in about 9 p.m. and drag my luggage to the third floor room. It was a very nice suite but was missing a minibar. There was no hotel restaurant, and more importantly, there was no hotel bar!

I had nothing to eat since breakfast, so I ordered a pizza for delivery. I then took a brisk, frigid walk in 10 degree weather to a neighboring Hilton Hotel to purchase two bottles of wine at inflated prices. I certainly had no intention of flying off to Liberia and catching Ebola without a good glass of wine first.

At 8 am the next morning I trotted down to the hotel lobby to await pick up by Annie, the ARC Human Resources Coordinator. Two young men were waiting in the small lobby, each carrying backpacks. I asked if they were waiting for Annie, and I met Mark, a nurse from St. Louis, and Jonathan, an ER nurse from rural Montana. They would both be on our Ebola Emergency Response Team to Liberia and had previous international healthcare experience.

I immediately liked them both. They were young, energetic, and enthusiastic. As an older, more jaded soul, I have a lot to teach them.

Annie arrived in an SUV, and she was exactly how I imagined her, cute and vivacious. We drove to ARC headquarters as we made small talk about our individual trips to Minneapolis. The ARC headquarters is an old red brick building that has been beautifully restored with light wooden floors and modern, open offices and meeting rooms.

We gathered in a large meeting room to begin our orientation. I met Cher, an ER physician from Minneapolis, who was the other recruited doctor besides me. She was also newly retired, and like me was looking forward to making a difference in Liberia.

I also met Kelsy, a physician assistant (PA) from Minneapolis. Kelsy had been working in a workers' compensation clinic for several years and wanted to try something entirely different. She has come to the right place.

There were four nurses who had moved to Minneapolis from Liberia many years ago for better lives and careers: Isaac, John, Doris, and Demenia. Isaac was young, single, and smiled a lot. John was older, about my age, with four daughters and a wife. He worked as a nursing supervisor in a senior residency center. Demenia would be our medical coordinator, and Doris would be a nurse manager along with Jonathan.

In total, there were nine of us at this first meeting of the ARC Ebola Emergency Response Team that would be going to Fish Town to initially staff and set up the ETU. Other team members would join us once we settled in Fish Town. They included a medical director who was currently in quarantine from her last deployment to Liberia, lab and pharmacy personnel, and a dozen other Liberian nurses.

We had a full day of lectures regarding the history, science, and epidemiology of Ebola followed by talks detailing the treatment options available in rural Liberia where we would be practicing. There is no specific antiviral medication for Ebola. Treatment is aimed solely at controlling the effects of Ebola, which are primarily dehydration and shock from the inevitable vomiting and diarrhea that occur during the illness. We could treat the dehydration using oral rehydration therapy and/or peripheral IV fluids. There would be no lab for measuring electrolytes, liver, or renal function. There would be no blood products, oxygen, or ventilators available. There would be no supplies for central line insertion to measure intravascular volume and pressures. This would call for more of the art of medicine rather than the science.

There was another day of lectures regarding security, communication, media relations, quarantines, stress management, and coexisting with others in tight, adverse environments. Since I was an expert in all of the above, I dozed through most of the lectures. We also signed a contract to have no sexual relations for the duration of our trip. Am I going to Africa or a monastery?

On our last night of orientation, Jonathan, Mark, and I went to dinner at a nearby restaurant. We talked about our upcoming adventure and made a toast together. Secretly, we were all thinking that someone in our group was going to die of Ebola. Let's hope it's not the old guy.

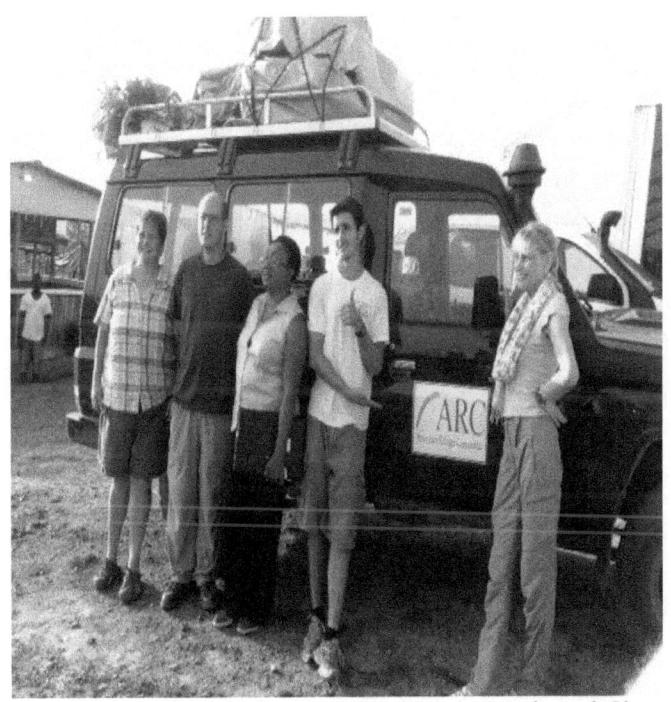

(From left to right) Kelsy, Jonathan, Doris, Mark, and Cher.

Dropping In

November 20, 2014

I awoke at 6 am to shower, finish packing, and grab a quick breakfast before hauling my luggage and backpack down to the lobby to wait pick up by a shuttle bus to the Minneapolis Airport. I was joined by Jonathan and Mark who had half the luggage I did. Obviously, they did not realize the importance of having six pairs of shoes available for daily dress at all times.

We arrived at the airport and met up with the rest of our medical group. As we approached the reservation desk, we were engulfed by local news media, consisting of a CBS affiliate with a cameraman and reporter along with a reporter from the Minneapolis Public Radio station. Many pictures were taken of us loading and checking our gear, and several of us were interviewed.

Reporter:"What does it feel like to fly off into certain death?"
Me: "Umm...good?"

After passing through security, we waited at our gate for our connecting flight to Chicago. From there we would then go on to Brussels, Belgium, and eventually Monrovia, Liberia. Most of us were quiet and kept to ourselves as we texted and sent last minute e-mails to friends and family. In our orientation classes most of us confessed that growing silent was one of the ways we exhibited stress. You could hear a pin drop.

We flew to Chicago and had a 3-hour layover. Some of us ate at an Italian restaurant and learned a little more about each other. I momentarily thought I had lost my backpack and accidently grabbed a stranger's backpack earning me suspicious looks.

Our flight to Brussels was on a monster plane, and there were plenty of empty seats surrounding each of us. I shared a bottle of wine with Cher, popped an Ambien, and slept about 4 hours of the flight. I woke 20 minutes prior to landing in Brussels, gulped down some hot tea, and splashed some water in my face.

The Brussels airport was covered with thick fog and had a surreal appearance after a long flight and little sleep. We crawled over to the gate operated by Brussels Airlines and set up temporary camp. There was a café a few gates away, and I purchased a large life-sustaining coffee.

Our next plane was huge also, but this time it was packed with international aid workers flooding in for the Ebola crisis. The overhead bins were an alphabet soup filled with backpacks labeled with decals for MSF, CDC, WHO, UN, and other health care organizations. I sat next to a nurse from Uganda who worked for Doctors Without Borders and was entering Liberia for the first time. He was pleasant but not very talkative.

We stopped in Dakar after a 6-hour flight. We had been traveling for over 24 hours and still had another 2-hour flight to Monrovia. Dakar appears to be a city of millions, judging by the number and vastness of lights in the fading twilight. Many passengers got up and stretched their legs and arms as if preparing for athletic competition.

Our plane took off, and we were on the final leg of our journey. The stewardesses strolled the aisles passing out pamphlets that loudly proclaimed, "Welcome to Liberia!" with a prominent photo of the Ebola virus on the cover followed by a detailed description of all the symptoms of Ebola. The Liberia Department of Tourism definitely has its work cut out for it.

Next stop, Liberia.

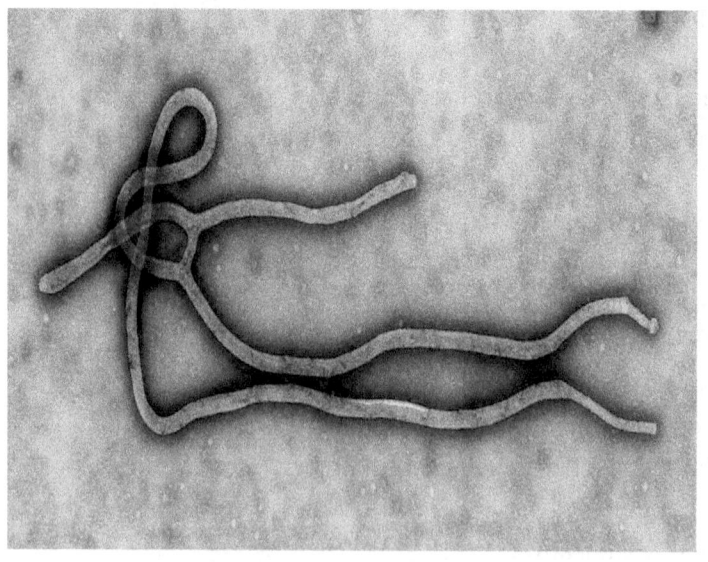

The Ebola Virus

Arrival Monrovia, Liberia

November 24th, 2014

Dear Friends and Family,

I awoke this morning to a beautiful voice talking in a near musical manner with low and high notes and ending her sentences with a laugh and a clap of her hands. I imagined she was telling a girlfriend about a boy she had just met. I opened the curtains and looked down two stories below me to a dirt alley. There was a woman in her 30s washing laundry by hand and speaking to a friend. The woman appeared happy with her life and without a worry or care.

We landed last night in Monrovia, the capital of Liberia, after 9 pm. We stepped out into the warm, humid air and were bused to the terminal. Before we could enter the terminal, we had our temperatures taken and were required to wash our hands under a stream of chlorinated water.

The terminal was packed with both returning Liberian residents and international health care workers. Standing in the long lines, I met individuals working with Doctors Without Borders, the CDC, and the United Nations. Many were returning to work in Ebola Treatment Units while some were new, like our group. Most of the individuals were young and single, but there were a few gray-haired individuals like me.

After about an hour of clearing customs, collecting our

luggage, and waiting for our ride, we were taken by private van and SUV to an apartment building. We are currently staying in two separate apartments with 3 bedrooms apiece. There is a spacious living/dining room, a kitchen, two bathrooms, and most importantly, AIR CONDITIONING! Did I mention that Liberia can be warm at times? Apparently, they are going to spoil us at first before putting us out in tents in the jungle for 3 months.

I am scheduled to do my hot/cold training next week starting Wednesday. It will be done in Bong County under the auspices of the International Medical Corp. The hot/cold training will last 7 days, and afterwards we will return to Monrovia to await deployment to Fish Town where our own ETU is under construction.

I attended a WHO Ebola overview meeting this morning. There were probably over a 100 individuals representing more than a dozen organizations. Dr. Francis, the Liberian Director of Health, spoke primarily about the epidemiology of Ebola and the plans to contain and eliminate it. He was touting the RITE plan (Rapid Isolation to Treat Ebola).

There were several Liberians who stood and spoke of the logistical problems of implementing the plan. Much of the country is jungle with difficult to near impassable roads, making it challenging to identify, transport, and isolate suspected or confirmed Ebola patients. Hopefully, with the massive influx of health care workers into the newly built Ebola treatment units, this will improve.

My coworkers are pleasant and thoughtful to be around. They come from a variety of different backgrounds in the health care field. When I have time, I will tell you about them individually. I suspect we will have plenty of opportunity to get to know each other over the next few weeks.

Love,

Joe

P.S. You cannot enter a store, hotel, or apartment without having to wash your hands first with chlorinated water.

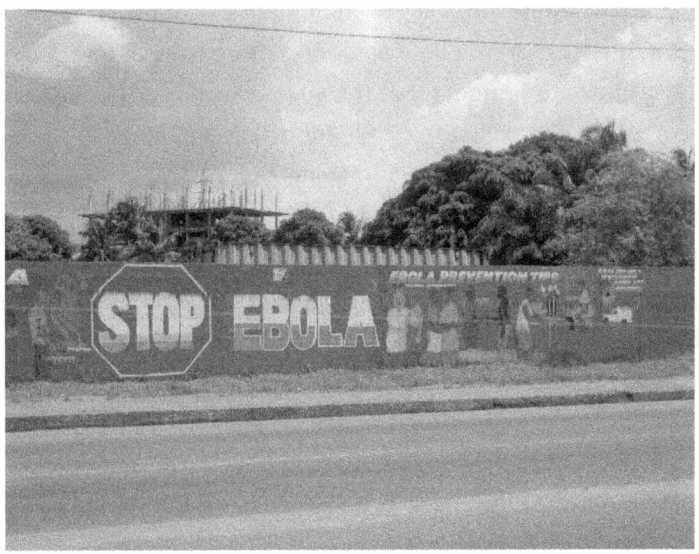

Informative wall in Monrovia, Liberia

Monrovia November 25th, 2014

Dear Family and Friends,

We are learning more about some of the cultural obstacles that have made control of the Ebola outbreak in Liberia so difficult. There is a deep distrust of the government by the Liberian people dating back for decades. This is due to a combination of two successive, bloody civil wars just ending in 2003, a long history of government corruption, and recent alleged fraudulent elections.

With the current Ebola epidemic, there have been widely circulated rumors that the government is poisoning the people and taking them to hidden places to harvest their organs to sell for profit. Imagine if you already distrusted the government and then you suddenly find newly built Ebola treatment units surrounded by fences and operated by strangers in costumes. Your family members are carted away by ambulances to enclosed tents to die. The body is then carried out wrapped in multiple bags so that your family cannot see the deceased. This has perpetuated the rumors, and much of the education of the Liberian residents has been to convince them that Ebola is real.

Another cultural obstacle that has been difficult to overcome is the tradition of Remembrance or Decoration Day. This is a national holiday typically held on the 2nd Wednesday in March to remember and honor the dead. Families go to the gravesites of relatives and have a party all day with food, drinks, music, and dancing. This is an important part of family tradition, much like Thanksgiving is for us. The initial cremation of Ebola victims by the government and health care workers outraged the public. They believe the body must be kept whole and buried in the family cemetery in order to continue the tradition.

The Liberian government has taken great steps in educating the public; although, the means of communication in Liberia are few. There is little television available, the Internet is hit and miss, and radio broadcasts are localized. Some of the best methods used to date are through the churches, county offices, and highway billboards. From looking at the latest declining Ebola numbers generated by the outlying counties and public officials, perhaps this is already starting to have an effect on stemming the tide of this awful disease.

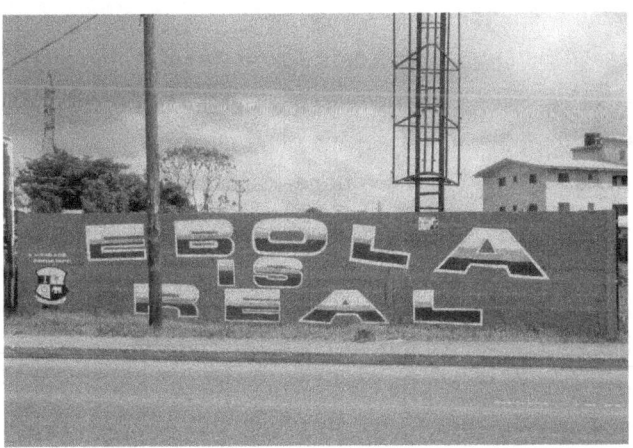

Painted wall in Monrovia, Liberia

Hanging Out in Monrovia

Dear Family and Friends,

Our team has had a couple of down days to rest up in Monrovia. We have traveled around the city on foot, in groups, and as individuals. The Liberian people are friendly, and the children enjoy waving at us. The public schools are cancelled due to the Ebola epidemic, so you see children out playing in the streets and yards every day.

The predominant mode of transportation in Monrovia is by motorcycle. Most often there are two riders on each motorcycle, and it is not uncommon to see 3 riders. The traffic patterns are erratic at best with no stop signs at most intersections, and cars and motorcycles weaving between and around each other.

To say Liberians like soccer is a gross understatement. There is a soccer field behind our apartment, and the men play from sun up to sun down. The older children play soccer in the street, and the younger children play in their yards. All day on Saturday people crowd around TV sets in the local bars to watch professional soccer.

The Liberians for the most part are very thin compared to the average American but amazingly strong. I saw two men carry a 250-pound safe up 2 flights of stairs the other day. The women carry large loads on top of their heads also. I saw a woman balancing a bowl on her head with 4 large fish hanging over the edges that must have weighed 40 pounds. I saw another woman with 4 chairs balanced on her head.

Saturday night we went out to eat at a local restaurant. The Liberian food is mainly white rice mixed with vegetables and either fish, chicken, shrimp, or beef. They use a local pepper to make a hot sauce that rivals habanero peppers in intensity and brings tears to my eyes. I can also report that the local Liberian beer (Club) is quite tasty.

There is a group of Russian helicopter pilots that live on the first floor of our apartment building. They pilot the UN helicopters that carry health care workers back and forth to Ebola Treatment Units (ETU) outside Monrovia. They have a statue of Vladimir Lenin on their front porch.

Late Saturday night, around midnight, we were out on our front porch talking when a UN truck came weaving down our street. It stopped in front of our apartment building and attempted to back up next to our perimeter wall. The truck accelerated at the last minute and crashed into the wall. It then pulled forward and slowly backed in, barely missing the adjacent car. The driver's door was so close to the nearby car that the driver had to slide out the passenger side. The driver spilled out onto the sidewalk, staggered through the security gate, fell down going up the landing steps, crawled to a first floor apartment door, and slithered inside. Our procurement manager, Walter, who has been staying here almost a month, diagnosed "too much vodka." At 6:30 am the next morning the UN truck was gone, the driver no doubt piloting a helicopter full of health care workers. I make a mental note to never ride in a UN helicopter.

Everywhere you go in Monrovia there are billboards advising against eating "bush meat," i.e. monkeys, rats, and fruit bats, that could be potential carriers of Ebola. Apparently, much of the BBQ you can buy on the streets is of unknown animal source. I have added BBQ to my list of things to avoid.

I attended a nearby Lutheran Church service on Sunday. It was similar in format to my own church in Austin. There was an all-women choir dressed in radiant, traditional dresses with matching headpieces. They sang and swayed to the beat of African drums.

The sermon was delivered in both English and Basso, a local language. It lasted more than 45 minutes and touched on a variety of issues but especially Ebola. Two community nurses walked down the church aisle, carefully scrutinizing the worshippers for signs of illness. Many people put their heads down on the pew in front of them during the Ebola portion in a prolonged prayer. Like my church in Austin, two men sitting next to me nodded off during the sermon.

A large portion of our group, including me, will be leaving for Bong County tomorrow to undergo cold/hot training in a busy, established ETU. It will take place over seven days and will include putting on the PPE (personal protective equipment) uniform, following the experienced doctors and nurses into the hot Ebola zones, and eventually participating in the care of the Ebola patients. I am looking forward to seeing my first Ebola patient since that is my primary mission here, but I feel guilty for doing so.

Road Trip to Bong County

Dear Family and Friends,

Our team arrived in Bong County late Tuesday night after a 5 hour van ride. Bong County is only 100 miles north of Monrovia, but the roads here are challenging. Imagine the worst semi-paved road you have ever driven on then carpet bomb it.

We had a delayed start from Monrovia when the rental van driver refused to drive us here. He thought we were just going to use the van to travel around Monrovia for the day and strongly objected to taking his van up to Bong. After an hour of negotiations and probably a bribe, we were able to proceed.

We drove out of the crowded city, and the landscape gradually changed to trees and fields rather than one-story shacks with metal roofs pressed tightly against each other. There was a continuous stream of humanity walking on the sides of the road with minimal clearance from the motorcycles, cars, trucks, and buses that rumbled by.

We came to some logs placed perpendicularly across our lane. We crossed to the other lane and drove by an area surrounded by logs. There was a covered body lying in the road with blood splatters surrounding it. We theorized that it was a pedestrian fatality rather than an Ebola patient. Apparently, such occurrences are frequent in Liberia. Another group at our training class had made the same drive in the morning. They told us that they saw the same body 6 hours earlier.

The landscape was interesting with gently rolling hills, scattered trees, and grasslands. There were giant ant mounds that approached 6 feet in height. We passed through frequent small villages that usually had a crowded marketplace and gas stations with clusters of motorcycle riders hanging around them. While passing through one village, we almost hit a little girl who dashed across the road to join her family

After a while we entered a landscape that had been deforested and planted with rubber trees. I was told that Firestone Tire and Rubber Company had leased thousands of acres here for decades. The Firestone Company built its own compound for processing the rubber and housing the workers and their families. The company even offers schooling and health care that is far above average for Liberia. They had a few cases of Ebola early on in the epidemic but immediately closed the compound to outside traffic and prevented any further cases. Their health care workers donned the protective gloves and aprons used by the rubber workers and they were not infected. The few initial patients either died or recovered. There are now guards posted at the entrance to the Firestone compound, and only approved groups or individuals are allowed in.

About 3 hours into our journey, the driver pulled over to the side of the road and stopped. He got out and announced a "rest stop." There were no visible buildings anywhere in sight. The men went out behind the van, and the women went in front. I likened it to an Oklahoma highway picnic area where there are no restrooms, just trails leading out into the woods.

As we traveled along we wove back and forth across the road to avoid giant potholes. We were passed on both the right and left sides by motorcycles and cars announced by much horn honking. As night fell the driver turned on his hazard lights but not his full beam lights. I am not certain what the advantage of this is, (less electrical drain? less gas?) but it does make for terrifying travel when you can only see about 10 feet in front of you. We narrowly missed colliding with several motorcycles and cars doing the same.

We finally arrived at our destination, Cuttington University in Bong County, about 8 p.m. We were directed to the women's and men's dormitories. They are single story and constructed of concrete blocks. We were given individual rooms with bunk beds. We sleep on the bottom bunk that is enclosed with mosquito netting that hangs from the upper bunk. There is a large shared bathroom with commodes and cold-water-only showers. There is no air conditioning, but we are each given an electric fan to use. My bed has a "Hello Kitty" bedspread, which is always a good sign.

The Bong County ETU is staffed and operated by the International Medical Corp, and they will be providing our training this week. There are 4 men and 4 women in our group, and we will be joined by other groups who are also training for soon to be opened ETUs. It is a mixture of doctors, nurses, and sanitation aids who will all be working in the high-risk Ebola treatment areas. Many countries are represented including Kenya, Uganda, England, and the United States.

After unpacking we ate dinner out of Styrofoam containers and prepared for bed. Shortly after retiring, there was a knock on my door. I opened the door and met Dr. Dziwe, the training director, and Audrey, a nurse and training coordinator. They introduced themselves, and we made small talk. After a few minutes, they told me that I should be aware of a certain situation that had developed.

There was an employee who was fired after he wrecked an International Medical Corp vehicle and was found to have drugs in his possession. The local police came and arrested him, but the prisoner escaped. He returned to the Cuttington campus and had a possible exposure to an Ebola patient in the process. He was briefly captured by the campus security but escaped again. He was subsequently seen lurking around the buildings where we are staying and training. Campus security guards have been placed at the entrances of our dorms. I was advised to lock my bedroom door and report any suspicious persons. He is described as 6 feet tall and goes by "Sunshine." It looks like it should be an interesting week here.

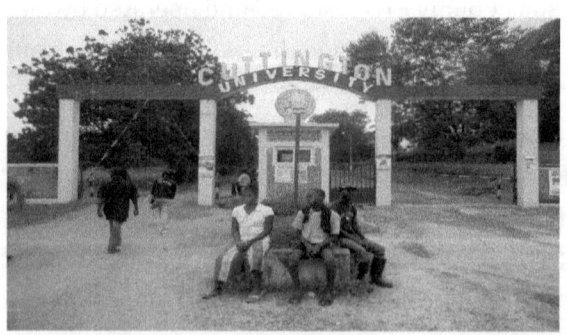

ETU Training Begins

Dear Family and Friends,

Our ETU training will last seven days divided into "cold" and "hot" sessions with the later being performed in an operational Ebola treatment unit. We will initially do three days of cold training where we will have lectures in the morning regarding the history, pathology, epidemiology, and treatment of Ebola. In the afternoon, training will be conducted on an outdoor basketball court with a mock ETU building. There we will practice putting on (donning) the PPE uniforms, triaging patients, starting IVs, drawing blood for Ebola testing, and removing (doffing) our PPE uniforms.

The lectures are given mostly by Audrey, our training coordinator. She is an excellent speaker and knows her material well. She has been working at the Bong County ETU for over 3 months. She has an infectious laugh and does not seem to mind the numerous questions we have for her. We also have a few lectures from doctors, epidemiology experts, and psychosocial workers.

I am particularly interested in the Ebola treatment recommendations gathered over the last several months by the different health care organizations such as Doctors Without Borders, International Medical Corps, and WHO. I am here to hopefully give effective treatment to the Ebola patients, and I would like to know what works and what doesn't work.

Oral hydration is the initial step in the treatment of all Ebola patients. A special electrolyte solution that contains a mixture of sodium, potassium, and magnesium is used. The patients are encouraged to drink a minimum of 1.5 liters of hydration fluid a day. We were given packets of the powder to pour into water bottles to sample. As you might expect from a flavorless solution containing potassium and salt, it has an unpleasant taste that I would have difficulty consuming in large quantities.

If the patient is severely dehydrated, as most Ebola patients will eventually become from all the diarrhea and vomiting, an IV can be started. This is obviously a delicate procedure since it involves sharp needles and direct contact with the patient. Extensive instructions were given on the correct way to do so. Patients are given 250-500 cc boluses of IV fluids containing sodium chloride and potassium over 1-2 hours since that is about the length of time a nurse or doctor can tolerate the heat while wearing the PPE uniforms.

Fluid input and output are estimated from whatever fluid (vomitus or diarrhea) ends up in the patient's bedside buckets. There are only two lab tests available: the Ebola virus test (an amplified viral load by PCR) and a malaria screen. No tests for electrolytes, kidney function, blood or platelet counts are available.

There is a standard protocol for febrile Ebola patients admitted to the ETU. They will receive a broad-spectrum antibiotic for 5 days along with an antimalarial medicine for 3 days. They also receive either Prilosec or Tagamet (drugs to protect the stomach) given the high incidence of vomiting and bleeding from the stomach. A multivitamin is given along with a zinc supplement. Oral potassium is available. Anti-nausea medications are given for vomiting or hiccups, a frequent occurrence in Ebola patients. Valium is used for mild agitation and Haldol for severe agitation. Confusion and delirium are common in the final stages prior to death. Tylenol is given for fever greater than 101. No intramuscular injections are given due to the bleeding abnormalities that occur in Ebola patients. Injections can cause large hematomas (collections of blood under the skin).

The donning and doffing of the PPE is both a physical and mental challenge. The training was conducted on a minimally shaded basketball court with a mock ETU unit building. It consisted of an enclosed tent with cots and separate donning and doffing areas. A step- by- step regimen of properly getting dressed and undressed was drilled into our heads.

The donning and doffing processes each take about 10– 15 minutes. You wear scrubs and rubber boots to begin with. All jewelry including rings, earrings, watches, and necklaces are removed. You climb into the PPE suit that provides the outer layer of the uniform covering your boots and extending upwards to your entire neck, much like a turtleneck shirt. There is a zipper in the front and several tabs on the uniform that have adhesive strips to tape the uniform over the zipper and around your neck. Three pairs of surgical gloves are put on with the last pair being fastened to your sleeve with duct tape. A duck -billed type surgical mask is put on covering your nose and mouth, followed by a complete headpiece with a second mask that overlaps the duck-billed mask. A hole is made in the outer mask, and the bill of the underlying mask is allowed to protrude outwards. A heavy apron is then donned in front and tied behind you by an assistant, leaving a free end on the side that can be pulled in the undressing process. Finally, a large pair of plastic goggles is placed over your eyes, making sure that no skin is exposed either on your forehead or cheeks. The overall look resembles a *Star Wars* Imperial Trooper, but instead of a man, you are a duck.

Movement in the PPE uniform feels clumsy and restricted. Wearing rain boots, a heavy apron, constricting clothes, and headpieces, I was worried that I was going to panic since I am a tad on the claustrophobic side. (I cannot stand to wear turtleneck sweaters normally because I feel like I am being choked). Combine that with the heat, humidity, and fear of contamination, and you have a recipe for panic attacks. I used mental imaging to project myself to a cooler location, such as Barton Springs Pool, to calm my nerves.

My anxiety situation was not helped by discovering two tears in the sleeve of the first PPE suit I put on with my skin visible underneath. The instructor examined the tears and stated that these were the first manufacturing defects she had ever found in these particular suits. A single opening could allow the Ebola virus to make contact with skin and potentially result in death. I made a silent promise to myself to examine all future PPE suits for defects before entering the ETU compound.

We walked through the mock ETU, looking at the beds,

mannequins, buckets, and hand wash stations. It was warmer in the ETU tent, and there was no breeze. It was about 85 degrees outside; adding the PPE uniform probably added another 5-10 degrees. I felt sweat running down my face and back.

Finally, we were done with the mock ETU tour and moved to the all-important doffing station. This is the most important step in preventing Ebola contamination in the healthcare worker. One by one we first stepped into buckets with chlorine solution and then moved forward to a red line painted on the asphalt. There was a sprayer who sprayed chlorine solution from front to back, including the arms, hands, and everything below the shoulders. We washed our hands in chlorine solution and then removed our outer gloves. We washed our hands again and then untied our aprons and placed them in a nearby receptacle. More washing of the hands was followed by removal of the goggles, being careful to not allow any moisture to hit our eyes or skin. We then untied three ties that secured our headpiece and one more tie across the chest. Then we bent forward and removed the hood by grabbing it behind our head and pulling it off.

The PPE suit itself is removed by opening the adhesive closures, unzipping, and then pulling the suit off your body without touching the outside. It involves a fair amount of body wiggling and resembles a very awkward strip tease. The duck-billed surgical mask is then removed followed by the second pair of gloves. Next, our boots are sprayed front, sides, back, and bottom, and we are allowed to step over the red line. The final pair of gloves is removed, we wash our hands a few more times, and we are finally done.

After 45 full minutes of wearing the PPE uniform, most participants found their scrubs soaked in sweat from top to bottom. We were given cold sodas to drink along with a liter of water. I felt mildly dizzy at one point and sat in a chair in the shade with a breeze. Despite drinking another liter of water, it was over 4 hours later before I could even urinate.

We practiced the PPE donning and doffing exercises for 3 days. On the 3rd day we discussed what to expect when entering an ETU with actual Ebola patients. We should never enter the ETU alone. We will always have someone with us, a "buddy". Do's and don'ts are reviewed: don't touch your goggles or face while in the ETU, don't allow any sharp objects to be pointed towards you or your buddy, always wash your hands between patients, and try not to touch any body fluids or surfaces while in the ETU.

After 3 days of cold training, we are ready for the next step. Tomorrow we will travel 3 miles to the Bong County ETU and begin our hot training. Our team has a meeting, and we discuss the fear that lies shallow in every one of us. The fear of Ebola, the fear of failure to perform our assigned tasks, and the fear of the unknown are discussed. We provide emotional support to each other and decide that courage is what it takes to move forward in our mission to help the Liberian people with this terrible disease.

Let it begin.

Love,

Joe

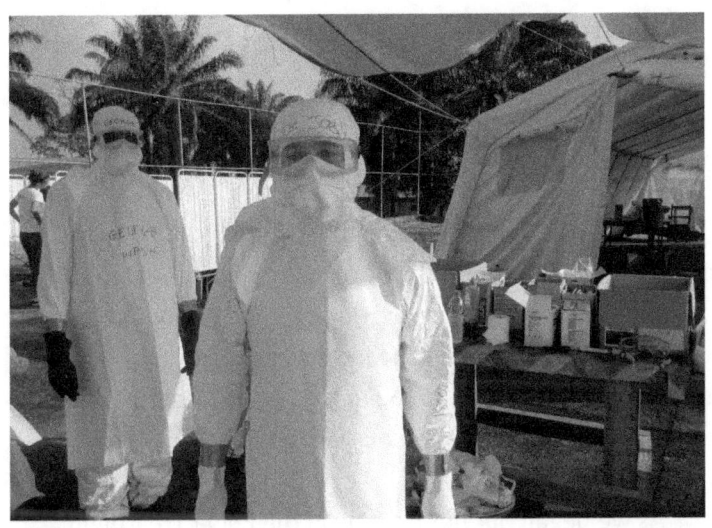

Dr. Joe in full PPE

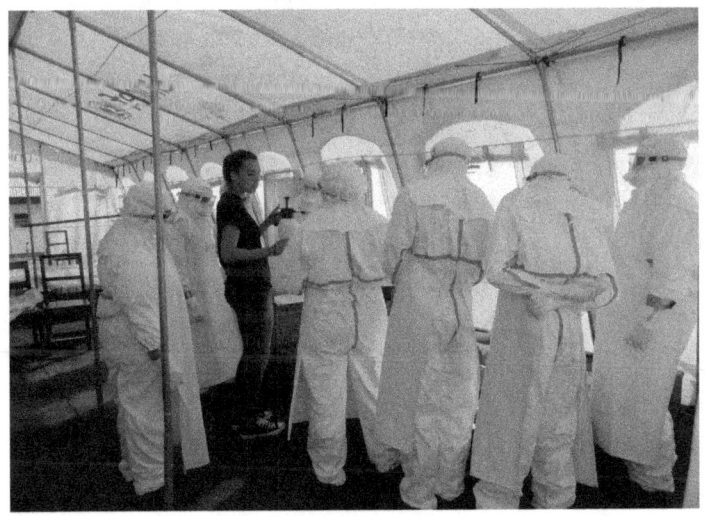

Training in the mock ETU

Hot Zone Training in the Bong County ETU

Dear Family and Friends,

The Bong County Ebola Treatment Unit is built on the site of a former Leper colony. It sits on top of a cleared hill with beautiful views of the jungle and distant mountains. It was the only location that the local population and authorities could agree on. Having an Ebola treatment unit in your neighborhood is obviously not a boost to home values.

As we began our hot training in the Ebola Treatment Unit (ETU), we were told that there are no real emergencies in the ETU. If a patient arrests, starts hemorrhaging, goes into labor, develops seizures, or quits breathing, we do not rush in to assist them. This was attempted early on in the epidemic with several medical worker fatalities.

MSF (Médecins Sans Frontières, aka Doctors Without Borders) who have treated more Ebola patients than any other group here has a motto for treating Ebola patients: "We are never in a rush to die", words to stay alive with.

On the first day our group of four arrived by bus shortly after noon. It was a blazingly hot day with much sunshine and little breeze. We passed two 4x4 pickups that were parked just outside the gate. The beds of the trucks were enclosed with plastic tarps and a plastic covered mattress was on the bed floor. These were the Ebola ambulances that transported patients from outlying areas. I imagined what it would feel like to ride in the back of the pickup if you were sick. Knowing the horrible Liberian roads, if you didn't have nausea and vomiting when you climbed in, you would by the time you arrived.

We were shown around the ETU with its changing rooms, offices, and donning and doffing stations. It was a beehive of activity with many Liberian workers constructing an additional water tower and another doffing station to handle the large number of healthcare workers and patients. There were two loud gasoline generators running to supply electricity to the ETU. An incinerator used to burn contaminated material was blowing a thick plume of black smoke at the back of the compound.

The first day we were given a tour of the suspected and confirmed wards. After donning the multilayer PPE outfits, we entered the hot zone of the ETU. It was separated from the rest of the compound by two rows of orange webbed plastic fences. Suspected cases are those patients who have been admitted with symptoms of Ebola, such as fever, headache, or vomiting. They will be tested for the virus and observed. Confirmed cases are those patients who are receiving treatment after testing positive for the virus. They are kept strictly apart since many of the suspected patients will turn out to be negative for Ebola and have malaria or some other illness.

The two suspected patients we saw appeared to be doing well and their fever and symptoms had resolved with empiric antibiotics and antimalarial treatment. They already had one negative Ebola virus test but would be retested in

48 hours.

The Ebola virus test measures the viral load in the bloodstream and often, early on in the infection, the test cannot pick up lower levels of virus. If the repeat Ebola test is negative, patients are discharged and told to return if symptoms reappear.

The confirmed ward had about 10 patients. Most were lying on their beds in the sweltering heat and appeared exhausted. A few conversed with us, but many were quiet and seemed to want to be left alone.

The sickest one was Victoria, a 22 –year-old female who was admitted 2 weeks previously with severe dehydration and fever. She was started on IV fluids and antibiotics, but a few days later developed seizures, stiff neck, and decreased mental status. Her seizures were treated with IV Valium 10 mg every 8 hours, and she was started on IV antibiotics for possible meningitis. No CT scan or lumbar puncture was done. Amazingly, she had improved, and was now sitting up, eating, and following commands. Her Valium was stopped, and she was now seizure free.

The staff discussed how long to continue the antibiotics, assuming she even had bacterial meningitis. Seizures are a known complication of the Ebola virus, but the etiology is unknown. Encephalitis? Viral meningitis? They decided on 7 days as long as she continued to improve.

Victoria had a rash on her right flank that we examined. It extended from under her right arm down to her waist in a fairly straight line with a sizeable area of skin denuded that looked like a burn or abrasion. The staff hypothesized that it could be due to prolonged bed rest or perhaps Nairobi flies that are common around here.

Since arriving, I have seen several of the nurses and doctors with erythematous facial streaks due to chlorine spray inadvertently hitting their face when doffing. I offered up the idea that perhaps the patient was accidently sprayed with or laid in the more potent chlorine solution that is used to clean the floors and rooms of the Ebola treatment areas. One of the staff doctors looked at me and diplomatically called my idea "interesting", i.e. bullshit. I felt like a 3rd year medical student first arriving on the hospital floor.

Many of the confirmed patients were in fact getting better and could possibly be discharged in a few days. Criteria for discharge from the confirmed ward includes:
1) no fever or gastrointestinal symptoms for 3 days
2) can feed, wash, and walk by themselves
3) a negative Ebola virus test.

Discharged patients are given fresh clothes and a certificate stating that they have been treated for Ebola and are now cured. Early on, many Ebola survivors were shunned by their families and communities when they tried to return home. The certificates seemed to alleviate this problem.

Men are told to not have sex for 3 months afterwards since their semen can still contain the Ebola virus for a prolonged period of time. They are also given condoms "just in case."

We were told that two weeks earlier they had over 40 patients in the confirmed ward, and they were having a death every day. The epidemic appears to have settled down, but it could blow up quickly given the infectivity of the virus.

After our tour of the facility, we were led by our guide to the outside of the compound and followed a trail along the side. We passed the morgue and a two wheeled, elongated cart that is used to transport the dead bodies. We followed a narrow winding trail that led us away from the ETU and into the jungle. As we walked along, the sounds of the generator and workmen faded, and soon all we could hear were birdcalls and the wind rustling the leaves of the trees.

After about 200 yards we entered a small clearing and saw the graveyard. There were rows and rows of small white crosses with the name, date of birth (sunrise), and the date of death (sunset). Most are in their 20s, 30s, and 40s, but there were several young children and teenagers also. Many of the deceased were related to one another since one family member will tend to infect another.

The sight of this elicited silence and reflection in our group. There were perhaps 150 people buried here since the unit opened in September 2014. Along the edges were freshly dug graves awaiting the next victims. The graves were very precisely made, exactly 6 feet deep and 3 feet wide. The body of an Ebola victim is extremely infectious and can remain infectious for up to 3 months. Part of the difficulty in controlling the Ebola outbreak has been the cultural practice of bathing and touching a body prior to burial. Much public education has been put in place to stop this practice, but it is slow to change.

I met a gravedigger one day and spoke with him. Each day he dug a grave using a pickaxe and shovel. He wished he did not have to do his job, but he said he does it to show respect to the deceased and their relatives.

When a funeral occurs, families are allowed to follow at a safe distance while the body disposal team, dressed in full PPE, transports and lowers the body down into the grave. A worker follows the cart and sprays the ground with chlorine. A family member is allowed to place the cross, and a few words are said over the grave. Most Liberians are Christians and, unfortunately, have become very familiar with death.

One morning several blood draws needed to be done on the Ebola patients. I volunteered to draw one of the patients although I had not done so in years. We used a 23- gauge needle with syringe and were VERY CAREFUL since a contaminated needle stick guarantees an Ebola infection in just a few days. We used gloves for tourniquets because regular bands were not available. My hands were steady as I penetrated the vein, and I got an initial blood flash in the syringe. The patient grimaced and moved her arm, and the blood flow stopped. I tried to adjust the needle, but after a minute a hematoma started to form. I had blown the vein, and I knew it. I withdrew the needle and discarded it safely into the sharps box.

I was supremely disappointed, particularly so because a few of my teammates witnessed my failure to perform a relatively simple procedure. I decided to put it behind me and keep a positive attitude. Truthfully, in real practice, it is the nurses who start the IVs and draw blood. We have very capable nurses on our team, and I trust them to get the job done.

Much of the treatment of Ebola patients is empiric and conjecture. The lab and radiologic procedures we take for granted in the USA are nonexistent here. The doctors will go through the differential diagnostic possibilities and often pick a diagnosis based on the available treatment options.

One patient had a painful left knee and some increased swelling in her left lower leg. We examined the patient, and I believed she had a warm knee effusion and some stasis edema below it. Another doctor worried about a blood clot in the calf, even though there was no palpable cord and a negative Homan's sign. There was no ultrasound to confirm or rule out a blood clot. It hardly mattered since we had no Heparin or Coumadin to give. Even if we did, it would not be given since Ebola patients are prone to disseminated intravascular coagulation (DIC) with both bleeding and clotting going on at the same time. No joint aspiration could be done since we had no lab to process the fluid we would obtain. No NSAIDs or aspirin were given due to the high incidence of gastritis and bleeding. Joint complaints are common in Ebola patients and effusions have been reported in many. Once again, we decided on antibiotics for the effusion in case it might be a bacterial infection.

November 29th is a national holiday to celebrate the birthdate of William Tubman who is considered to be the greatest president of Liberia. There was a party going on at the local campus café, and Jonathan and I decided to attend. There were perhaps about 200 people gathered, nearly all Liberians, and Afro-Pop music was blasting out to scattered groups of dancers and revelers. Jonathan and I grabbed some Club beer and sat down to enjoy the show.

At the table next to us, we noticed a young woman who was one of the sprayers at the mock ETU drill. She smiled at us and toasted us with her beer. Next to her was a young man dancing very enthusiastically with a large beer in his hand and obviously quite inebriated. He tried to walk around us but crashed into our table, and our beers went flying. I made a great save on my beer, but some of it splashed on me. He apologized and staggered off to get another round. The young woman next to us shrugged her shoulders and smiled.

As we left and started back on the road to our dormitories, we saw multiple men in the field across the road relieving themselves. I decided to always walk on the roads from now on and avoid shortcuts through the fields.

The Internet has not been working here the past two days. The rumor is that the people in charge did not pay last month's Internet bill, and it has been cut off. Liberians with local cell phones can still communicate with the outside world, but many foreigners are feeling isolated.

The breakfast this morning was particularly good. There was cold oatmeal, a wheat roll, and not one but two hot dogs! Hot dogs are the most common meat items served at meals. They are served bare without a bun, with a dollop of ketchup and mayonnaise on the side. I initially ate most of the hot dogs given to me but have now developed a deep aversion to them. My brother refers to hot dogs as "tube steak", and we often like to guess at the animal products used in their production: ears, snouts, lips, anal rings, tails, etc., basically any part of the pig that is not good enough for sausage. Another popular food served for breakfast here is spaghetti covered with a spicy, oily sauce. I tried it a couple of mornings but did not care for it. It must be an acquired taste.

There was a bucket in my dorm room that I assumed was for trash and used it as such. One day I took the full bucket out to the hallway to be picked up by the janitors and discovered, much to my horror, that others had also placed their buckets out in the hallway, but instead of trash they were filled with dirty laundry! I left my bucket full of trash out in the hallway for emptying, but it disappeared that afternoon and never returned. Apparently, I have lost my laundry privileges.

I have learned from talking to other U.S. doctors and nurses at the Bong County ETU that they are allowed 2 weeks of R and R every 6 weeks. I asked what was the point of going on vacation outside of Liberia if you would be required to stay at home for the 21-day quarantine. They informed me that England and Western European countries, such as Belgium, France, and Italy do not enforce quarantine on returning Ebola healthcare workers. This is an epiphany to me since I had thought that a 21-day confinement to my house in Texas on my return was the only available option. Instead of immediately returning to the U.S. after leaving Liberia, I could spend 21 days vacationing and traveling in Western Europe. Perhaps I could even talk June into joining me for an extended honeymoon for 3 weeks. I might even pop over to England to visit my good friend Russell Secker and check out the local pubs there. It would sure beat the heck out of returning to Texas and being locked up like Old Yeller to see if I go rabid and need to be put down.

I like to get up early in the mornings and walk around the campus. It is the coolest part of the day and the most peaceful. There is a bird here called the cuckoo bird that I often hear. Its call is an exact rendition of the Cocoa Puffs commercial "Cuckoo for Cocoa Puffs!" That must have been the easiest jingle ever created. There are also numerous flowers that open up in the morning, much like morning glories. One is particularly beautiful and resembles an iris or orchid.

One day we examined one of the ETU nurses who had a painful eruption on the back of his neck. There is a bug here called the Nairobi fly that doesn't actually fly but crawls. The Nairobi fly does not bite, but if purposefully or accidently smashed against your skin, a toxin is released from its body which causes an almost chemical-like burn over a large area. Multiple painful vesicles appear with what appears to be white pus in them. They will last for several days before eventually resolving, leaving a large denuded area of skin to slowly heal over the next couple of weeks. This particular nurse felt something crawling on him in the night and awakened with a searing sensation in the back of his neck. It started about 3 days ago and the vesicles are still visible with surrounding redness. He has been started on antibiotics to prevent a secondary infection.

We also visited the nearby US Navy lab that has been brought in to provide emergency Ebola virus testing for much of Liberia. It is operated by Navy PhD scientists specializing in highly pathogenic organisms such as Ebola, bird flu, Marburg, etc. Pathogenic viruses are ranked by level of infectiousness and deadliness with Level 1 being the least virulent and Level 4 the most. The Ebola virus is a Level 4 and requires expert handling and processing that only a few specialized labs can provide.

Ebola is a single stranded RNA virus that is protected by an outer coating. When a blood specimen is brought in, the scientists put on PPE uniforms and first deactivate (kill) the virus with chlorine and then alcohol solutions. After this process the virus is considered non-infectious and is transported to an extraction station. There the RNA is attached to DNA for better measurement. The remaining DNA is then amplified and measured based on the number of amplifications required to reach a standard level. If there is no RNA found from Ebola, it will be a flat line. It is said to be an extremely sensitive test and can pick up very low levels of virus, but there can be a lag time of several days between onset of patient symptoms and the ability to detect the virus. Some scientists have hypothesized that the virus is building up its troops in the lymphatic system prior to invading the blood stream.

On our last night here, we had a big party in celebration of finishing our training and making many new friends. One of the Liberian-American nurses had family nearby, and they brought in large quantities of fish, chicken, rice, and fruit. Jonathan and I supplied the beer, and a Kenyan worker brought in a karaoke program on his computer with a speaker. Soon we were taking turns singing various songs, many of them American. One man had a remarkable voice and could be a contestant on *American Idol* with sweet high and deep low notes. Another nurse is also a good singer. She does so with much emotion and gyrations of her body.

A particularly emotional and moving moment occurred when we all sang "We Are The World" together. It was a multinational, multiethnic group gathered on this night, and looking around the room, I saw people from Uganda, Kenya, Nigeria, Liberia, England, and the United States. We were the world coming together to fight Ebola.

One of the nurses brought in some local palm wine and sugar cane liquor. I sampled the wine, which is milky in color, and found it tart and nasty. I also sampled the sugar cane liquor which was clear and tasted like cheap tequila. Several of the nurses mixed it with sodas, drinking liberally. Judging by the effect it had on them, it also seemed to have the same results as tequila. The imbibing nurses were soon up singing and dancing with each other and trying to drag guys out on the dance floor. They tried to get me up, but I declined proclaiming, "Nobody wants to see an old white guy dancing," which elicited lots of laughs. One of the nurses kept asking, "Where is my Johnny?" over and over again. "Johnny" is apparently the common slang used for a boyfriend or girlfriend in Liberia.

Tomorrow we leave for Monrovia to have a few more days of cold training and to wait to hear when our Ebola Treatment Unit in Fish Town, River Gee will be completed. As with most things in Liberia, it is behind schedule and may not open until late December.

I feel confident that the training we have received here

is the best we could have. The Bong County ETU has a mortality rate of around 60% that, while still too high, is better than the 75 -80% mortality figures I have often seen quoted. The doctors and nurses here are truly saving lives with minimal resources. I am honored to have met and worked alongside them.

When our group arrived here last week, we were eight individuals still trying to get to know each other. After a week overcoming the fear and anxiety involved in the care of Ebola patients, we have met the challenges, both internal and external. We are returning a cohesive team, our sum being greater than the individual parts.

It's a good start.

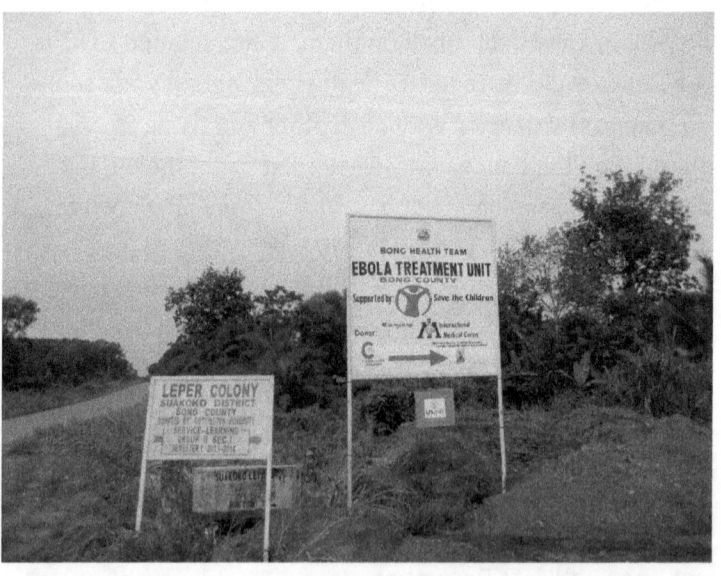

Signs marking entrance road to the Bong County ETU

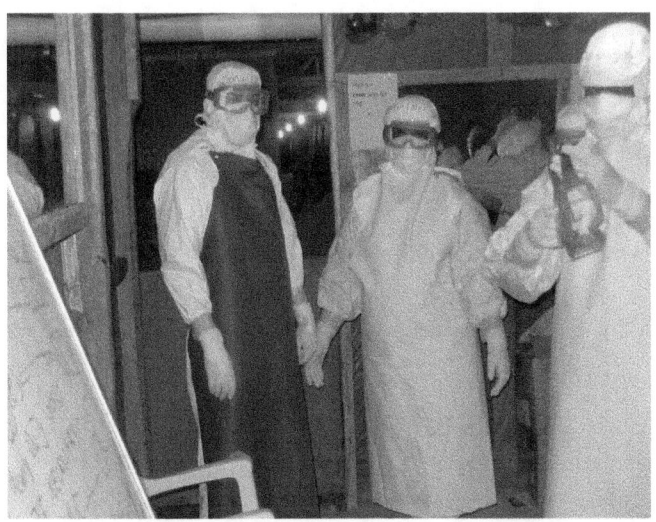

Jonathan and Minnie prepare to make ETU rounds.

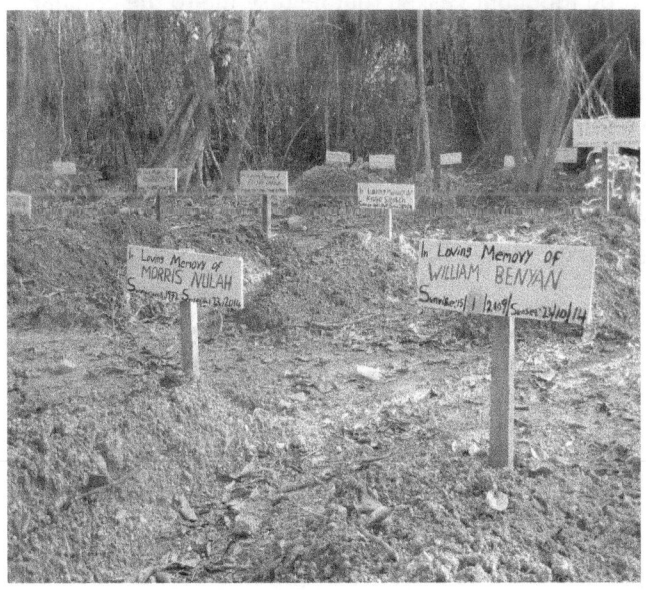

Bong County ETU graveyard

Random Stories from Liberia

Our group has two drivers who transport us around to meetings, stores, and other destinations. Both drivers are native Liberians and quite friendly. One afternoon I was going to walk to a nearby, recommended restaurant but was uncertain of its exact location. One of the drivers, Lawrence, offered to guide me.

We started off in the opposite direction than what I had planned, but I assumed he knew the way. After several blocks of walking, we arrived at an entirely different restaurant than where I had intended to go. He assured me it was good food, but I asked that he take me to the original restaurant I had requested. We walked around the neighborhood in a large circle, eventually returning to the same restaurant we were at previously. I realized that Lawrence was not going to lead me to my requested restaurant and agreed to eat at his restaurant choice.

When we walked in it was immediately apparent that Lawrence knew many of the staff in the restaurant. We sat down, ordered, and made small talk. He told me he knows Monrovia and Liberia better than anyone. If I ever needed anything, I should just let him know and he could find it.

As we started to eat our food, he pointed out a young woman at the bar and asked if I thought she was pretty. I glanced at the woman who was sitting on a bar stool and appeared bored. I replied yes, that she was pretty. He leaned over and said, "I can get her for you, good price. In Liberia prostitution is not crime."

I pointed out that: 1) I was married and   2) I did not wish to dodge Ebola only to die from HIV disease (rampant in prostitutes in Africa). Lawrence nodded his head and replied, "Yes, I understand. Perhaps I ask you again next week after you return from Bong County?" (Note to self: delete wife from Liberia e-mail group.)

The organization I am with is still trying to find a helicopter service to contract with for possible emergency medical evacuation from Fish Town in case someone in our group comes down with Ebola. Transporting Ebola patients is hazardous work and requires extensive viral hazard protection and decontamination afterwards. The transportation coordinators have been in touch with numerous private and public helicopter services but no takers as yet. It would take at least 2 days of bone jarring driving on the roads to return to Monrovia for intensive medical care. In Ebola time, you are dead.

I am reconsidering my position on UN helicopters and have purchased a bottle of vodka for a possible bribe to the Russian pilots downstairs, just in case.

One night Mark, Henry, and I went to a beach club that was far away from our apartment in Monrovia. We easily got a ride out to the club but would have to find our own ride back. It was a lively club with many Americans present. Many were attending a sendoff party for a comrade that had finished her deployment to Liberia and would be going home. We did not know the individual or group involved and sat at the periphery of the bar area, nursing our drinks and having dinner.

After dinner Henry joined a game of pool that he had been eyeing from a distance. Henry is a pretty good player, and the Liberians enjoy his company. We had intended to come home early, but the pool game escalated into a series of games, and before long it was approaching midnight. Henry and his partner won the final game on a terrific shot by Henry, and we were finally able to leave.

When we exited the restaurant there were no taxis to be seen. We asked the parking attendant if he could call a taxi for us, but he told us that if we just walked a few blocks out to a main thoroughfare, we would be able to hail a taxi easily.

So the three of us, two white guys and Henry, started walking down the side street a few blocks and eventually joined up with a busier avenue. During this time we were hailing taxis, but they were all full or off duty. We then started sticking our thumbs out in the universal language of hitching a ride.

Fifteen minutes went by as numerous vehicles passed us. Finally, when we were just about to abandon hope and start the long walk home, an SUV pulled over. Inside were two Liberians who were listening to Kenny Rogers' song, "The Gambler," blasting out of the stereo system.

The driver was friendly and offered to drive us all the way back to our apartment. We chatted as we rode along and thanked him for picking us up. He told us that initially, when he saw us on the side of the road, he wasn't going to stop. Why take a chance picking up white foreigners late at night in a big city? But after he saw the black guy with us, he decided it would be safe to do so. The table turns on the white guys.

The night before we left for Bong County to begin our hot and cold ETU training, Jonathan and I went out to dinner with two American public health nurses who would act as advisors for our group. One of the nurses was actually raised in Bong County as a young child of Anglo missionary parents. We inquired as to what to expect in Bong County.

She described a small, crowded town with a few bars and restaurants and many street vendors. She then went on to describe in vivid terms all the episodes of gastrointestinal disasters she had experienced in Bong County from eating the food and drinking the water.

Jonathan and I critically evaluated this new information and decided that the most effective use of our daily food per diem would be to spend it on beer. Our theory is that the Ebola virus cannot survive in 40 proof blood.

I was talking to a doctor from Kenya who trained with us in Bong County for work in another ETU. I told him we would be out in a very isolated part of Liberia where there currently were very few cases of Ebola being reported. We had talked in our team of going out into the community to meet the local tribal leaders and residents for educational purposes.

He cautioned me to be very careful. He reported that a small group of white doctors and nurses went to a village in Sierra Leone to pick up an Ebola patient, and they were attacked and killed by a small mob. There were still persistent rumors among rural villagers that the government was sending foreigners in costumes to capture people, take them to a secret location to harvest their organs, then poison and kill them. The doctor said it would be safer for me to have American-Liberians approach the community leaders first and engage their trust before I showed my face. I have a new moniker, "The White Devil."

In parts of Africa white people are commonly referred to as "Blands". When Jonathan and I were in Bong County, our names were occasionally switched by a few of the locals. Jonathan is 6 feet tall, half my age, wears glasses, and is balding on top. After a Liberian called me Jonathan for the second time, I politely corrected him. His excuse was "All you Blands look alike."

Liberia appears to be the final resting spot for all discarded or donated American T-shirts. You see everything from community swim team shirts to unknown rock bands. Often the T-shirts do not seem to match the person wearing them. I have seen a man with a pink Britney Spears shirt and another man wearing a Soccer Mom shirt. I passed a teenage Liberian boy today who was wearing a Texas Longhorns T-shirt. I flashed him a Hook 'em hand sign, but I don't think he understood. He was smiling, however, and I took that as a good omen.

We heard a story about a medical team in Sierra Leone that was captured by a rebel group in the backcountry. The rebels demanded money and goods from the foreigners, but the captive volunteers had very little on them. A physician assistant was pulled out of the group, had his hands tied behind his back and a hood placed over his head. He was threatened with decapitation if the group did not come up with more money. A rebel searching through his baggage found a stethoscope and showed it to his leader. The rebel leader then realized that his hostages were medical workers there to treat Ebola patients. The PA was immediately released, and the medical group was allowed to continue on its way. I have now started wearing a stethoscope around my neck, just in case.

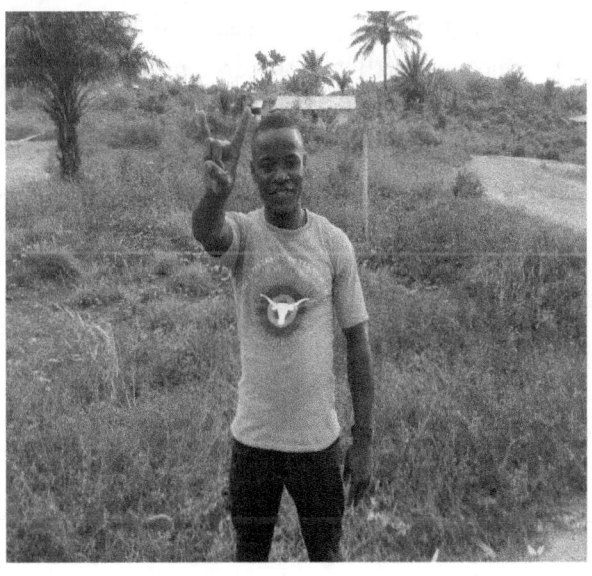

Texas Longhorn fan in Fish Town, Liberia

Shopping in Liberia

With only a couple of weeks now remaining in the Christmas shopping season, you are no doubt wondering, "Joe, what is the shopping like in Liberia?" You probably did not actually wonder that, but since I have nothing better to write about I will tell you anyway.

Need some quick snacks for those hungry guests and relatives that seem to always be hanging around? Go no further than your local open-air food market. A favorite treat for watching football games (soccer, not American football) is chicken feet!!! Yes, prepared properly chicken feet make a tasty snack for all.

If Americans are obsessed with chicken wings, the Liberians are likewise in love with the feet. And best of all, after stripping the delectable meat off the bones, you can use the claws as toothpicks! How great is that?
Raw fish and goat are also available for purchase.
Flies cost extra.

One afternoon I went fabric shopping with some ladies in our group. (Yes guys, I am that bored.) The fabric stores are packed into a few short blocks in downtown Monrovia. They are filled with hundreds of fabrics brought in from all over Africa, China, and India. The colors and patterns tend to veer towards the flamboyant side with bright reds, yellows, oranges, purples, and greens. Some are flat out gorgeous.

The ladies and I patiently combed through pieces of fabric and eventually found a couple that we mutually liked. The women immediately snatched up the fabric for purchase, leaving me empty handed. There were no duplicates of the fabrics, just one of a kind. We moved on to the next store, and the same thing happened again.

At the following store I was on my game and quickly grabbed a couple rolls of fabric. The asking price was $15 apiece. I attempted to bargain the price down but was unsuccessful and paid $30 for the two rolls. One of the ladies with me also had two rolls of similar fabric. The asking price was $15 apiece, but she got them both for $25 when she threatened to walk out.

I am a suckerfish out of water with these women.

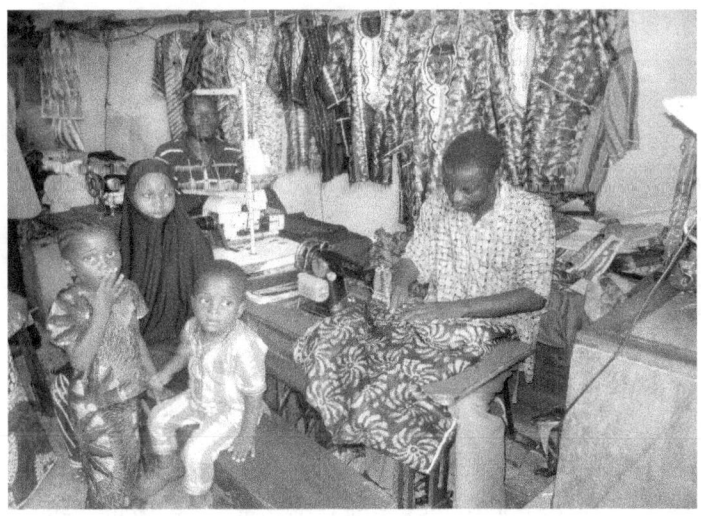

Getting a custom made shirt in Monrovia

Liberia Movie Reviews

I share an apartment in Monrovia with my teammates, Jonathan and Mark. They are both half my age but tolerate my presence. We often sit around at night over a few beers and discuss a wide range of subjects. One of the topics that invariably arises is the best movies we have ever seen.

Jonathan and Mark are great guys but have widely divergent opinions from me on cinema. Mark is convinced that *Road House* is the greatest movie of all time. The movie is about a bar in Missouri that has been taken over by a gang of thugs that work for a local crime lord, played by Ben Gazzara. Most nights the bar is open, the gang appears, gets drunk, molests the women, and tears the place up.

Patrick Swayze's character is brought in by the bar owner to bring order and control back to his bar. Patrick Swayze sports a mullet, speaks few words, and makes you wish you had never heard the words he does speak:
"It's my way or the highway."
"Expect the unexpected."
"I want you to be nice until it's time not to be nice."
He concludes with the immortal line delivered to a beautiful doctor in an emergency room who is sewing Swayze up, "Pain don't hurt."

Patrick Swayze is tight-lipped and occasionally adds a scowl, smirk, or nod to his acting repertoire. He exclusively wears tight T-shirts, showing off his muscle bound upper chest and arms. He is, of course, a martial arts expert (in addition to being a fabulous dancer as we saw in *Dirty*

Dancing) and uses both his arms and legs as lethal weapons. The whole movie is a string of fight scenes with Patrick Swayze beating the bejesus out of multiple bad guys until the final showdown with Ben Gazzara, the ultimate bad guy. The movie is a young man's wet dream of physical conquest and victory over evil.

I have tried to have a meaningful dialog with Mark and Jonathan about alternative cinematic productions that might be somewhat better than *Road House*. I have suggested classic comedies such as *Animal House* or *Caddy Shack* as appealing to a higher level of intelligence and comedic sense. I have also suggested *Gran Torino* or *Slum Dog Millionaire* as movies that would appeal to a greater sensitivity and morality than *Road House*.

My suggestions were carefully considered by both Mark and Jonathan but were ultimately rejected for lack of manly action and brutality. I have now decided to steer the conversation towards less controversial topics, such as religion or politics. Either that or I must find new roommates in Liberia who want to go fight Ebola. Good luck on that.

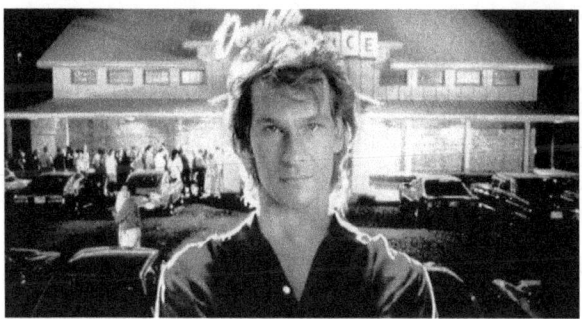

The Golden Beach Club

There are several beach bars and restaurants around Monrovia, but our favorite one so far is the Golden Beach Club. It is a long walk from our apartment (about 2 miles), and you work up a good thirst in the process.

There is a covered patio area in case it rains, but the premium tables are set out on the beach. The sand is fine and soft on the feet, and the surf is pleasant to watch and hear. The beach faces west, and there are great sunsets.

The Atlantic Ocean feels surprisingly cool, considering the tropical climate. Sadly, there is a lot of trash that washes up on the sand and subdues any desire to actually get in the water. There are also extremely strong rip tides that claim more lives than all the tropical diseases combined in Liberia. An engineer in our group told me that one day he saw a child's body wash up on a beach nearby. None of the locals would go after it, so he carried the body up to the street himself.

My friend George loves to have his picture taken on the beach. Every trip we make here involves a minimum of 50 pictures of George standing, squatting, sitting, and laying on the sand. When we return home George immediately downloads all the pictures of himself onto his computer. Afterwards, I go through the photos on my camera and delete 99% of them.

There are usually several tables of other aid workers from various countries at the Golden Beach Club. Russia, India, Canada, Pakistan, and Germany are well represented.

I see hookahs frequently being passed around at some tables. The Germans are the most vocal, drink the most beer, and are, no doubt, plotting their next attempt at world conquest. The Russians prefer vodka and are usually quietly studying the crowd for weaknesses.

The restaurant specializes in fresh lobster. For $24 you get a large grilled and cracked lobster with melted butter, salad, and French fries. I wasn't able to eat all of my meal and fed some to a rooster strutting around on the beach. I didn't know roosters liked lobster.

Usually around sunset, a man dressed in costume appears on stilts with a bongo player and commences to dance. He is said to represent the devil. The more money you place in his basket, the more frenzied his dancing. I am not sure if he is dancing for good luck or to place curses on your enemies, i.e. tax collectors, malpractice attorneys, ex-wives, etc.

Usually a fair amount of Club beer is consumed by the time we leave. We stumble through the sand past the tables of prostitutes and take a taxi home.

I realize that my behavior does not appear to be a very effective strategy to fight Ebola, and I apologize for that. I do go to the numerous daytime meetings covering the latest Ebola numbers, treatment strategies, up and coming vaccines, and antiviral medications under investigation. We have team meetings where we discuss how we would like our own ETU set up and organized. Until our ETU opens there is little we can do as a medical team. After 3 weeks in Liberia, we are all getting a little homesick and ready to move on.

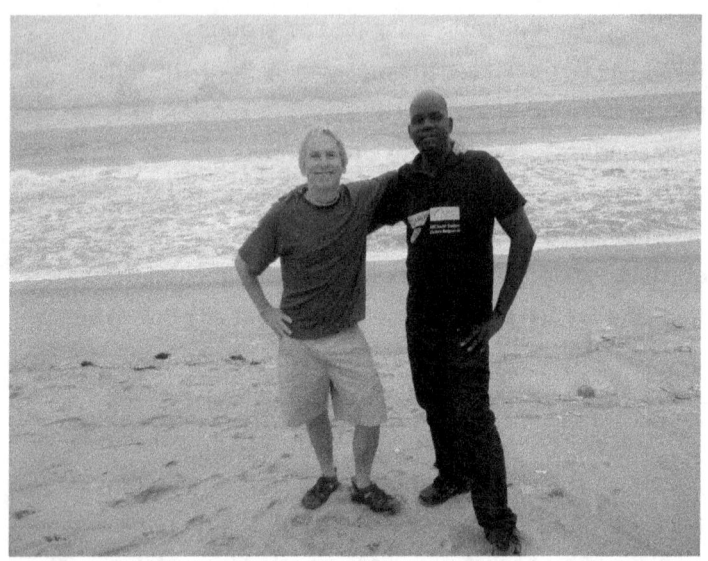

George and me at Golden Beach. George is on the right.

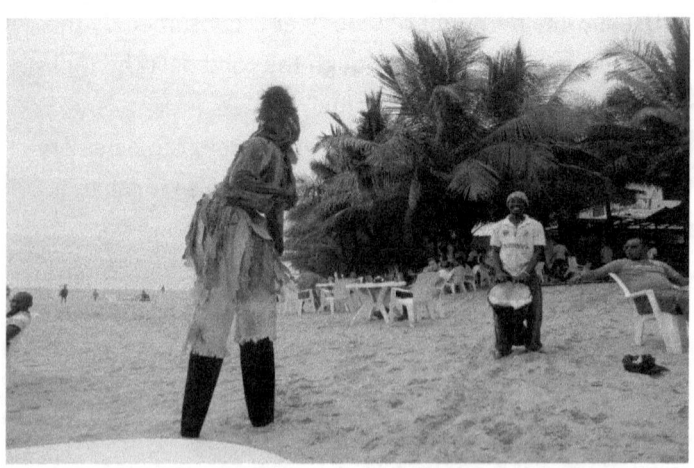

The Devil dancing at Golden Beach

Hurry Up and Wait

The only constants in Liberia are heat, humidity, and plans that change by the hour.

Two days ago I was told to pack my bags and prepare for a road trip to Fish Town. Then the departure date was pushed back a day. Later on I was told they had found a small plane that would fly us to Fish Town on Friday.

I reluctantly agreed to fly, although, I hate small planes where I can see the pilot drinking coffee while pointing out interesting geographic features far below us instead of watching where he is going. I see the hundreds of mysterious dials, lights, and controls moving and flashing ominously and anticipate eminent disaster at any moment. I usually have a death grip on my armrests and read the directions to the vomit bag repeatedly. I sure hope they have cocktail service on the plane.

The night prior to my scheduled 7:30 am plane flight, I was notified about another change in plans. I had been bumped from the plane, and I was now back to the original two day road trip, which would leave Saturday in a caravan of four-wheel drive vehicles. It remained unclear as to which other members of our team would be going with me.

We were told that our ETU in Fish Town was nearly completed, but our tents were still in Sweden awaiting transport. There has been a large influx of people and medical supplies into Liberia the past few weeks, and the already limited incoming plane flights have been overwhelmed. The priority has been to get the ETUs up and running as quickly as possible, which is the right choice. Building the housing for the healthcare workers (in our case large tents) will have to wait, so there is a problem of where to put the healthcare workers in the meantime. They tell us that a guest house has been rented in Fish Town in the interim. I interpret this as a bed and breakfast in a Victorian style with canopied beds and lace doilies everywhere. Our procurement manager, Walter, who has actually been there, just rolled his eyes and laughed. Not a good sign.

Since this was the last night for me in Monrovia for a while, we went out to Fuzion, an upscale bar and restaurant. The guys spotted a special cocktail on the menu, the Smokey Joe, and ordered one for me. It has tequila and lime juice and comes with a cute little umbrella, signifying a quality drink.

As usual, there were some prostitutes hanging out at the bar. Henry and I joke a lot about all the "pretty girls" we see around such places. Henry is in his 30s, married with kids, and doesn't drink alcohol.

There was a pool table in the corner. Henry walked over and was soon playing a game with a local. About three games later, Henry took a bathroom break, and when he returned his fellow pool player had invited two prostitutes to play with them.

Both girls were wearing the standard "hooker" uniforms of low cut tops and short, tight skirts with high heels. When they leaned over the pool table to take a shot, there was a lot of exposed flesh of which moms and wives all over the world would universally disapprove.

I could see that Henry was feeling uncomfortable with the unfolding situation, and he exited after playing only one game with the ladies. I offered to take a picture of him with the pretty girls to send to his wife. That earned me an icy stare. What a grouch.

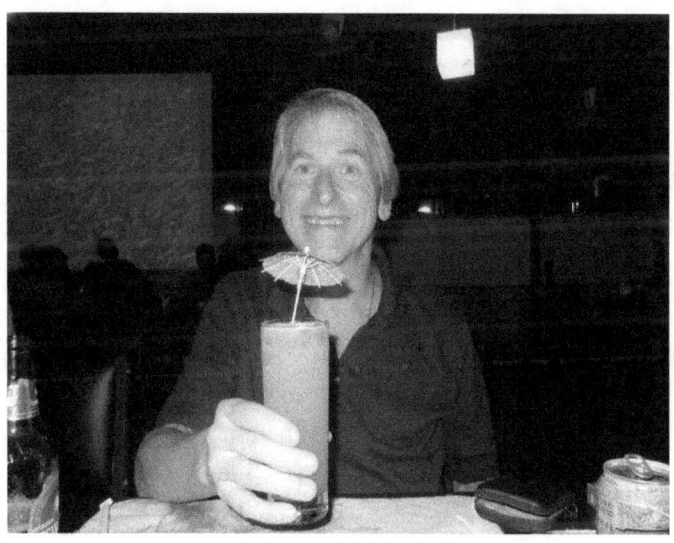

Dr. Joe meets Smokey Joe

Off to Fish Town

Dear Family and Friends,

It will take us two days to travel 350 miles on the torture devices that pass for roads here. I will be the first doctor from our group in Fish Town. I would like to think I was chosen because I am the most experienced, but Jonathan assures me it is because I am the most expendable.

I will be evaluating the layout and functionality of our brand new Ebola Treatment Unit (ETU). Of course, all I know is what I saw in Bong County during my training a couple of weeks ago. I will do my best to at least act like I know what I am doing. It wouldn't be the first time I have done so in my medical career.

Today I am going grocery shopping with Ade, our cook. We will prepare a feast for our medical team and support staff. I am hoping to find some big red snappers to grill, fry, and bake. Some fresh shrimp and crab would be nice also. It may be the last night we have together for a week or more. The rest of our team may not join me for a while.

I am looking forward to moving on to Fish Town and beginning the next chapter in my Liberian adventure. We have been told there have been no Ebola patients in River Gee County for the past 3 weeks. If that data is correct (all Ebola numbers gathered by the local counties are questionable), then that would be good.

Of course, I would like to use my medical skills and new knowledge for treating Ebola patients but not at the expense of human suffering. I have been told there is presently no Internet service in our ETU. In fact, there is no electricity yet because the generators are not in place. There may be an Internet café in Fish Town proper, 3 miles from our ETU, that I may be able to use. I'll find out when I get there in two days.

Love,

Joe

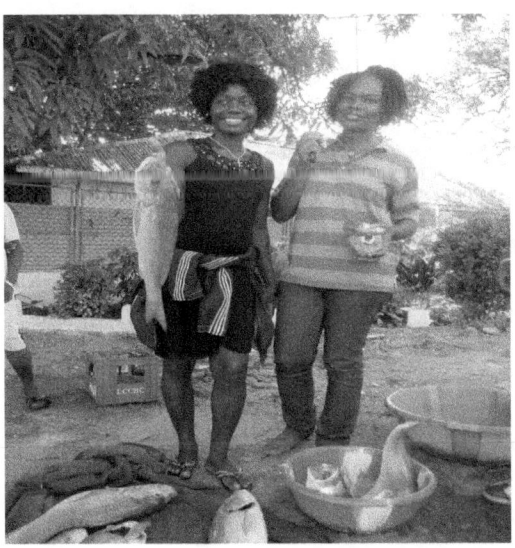

The best cook in Monrovia, Ade (in striped shirt),
standing next to woman holding large red snapper

Road Trip to Fish Town

Dear Family and Friends,

Departure day I awoke at 6 am to finish packing and gulp down some hot tea and a Red Bull. I pulled my luggage down two flights of stairs to the outside parking area for pickup at 7:30 am. At 8:30 the truck finally pulled up and loaded my luggage. We drove the two short blocks to our office compound where the first wave of our medical team was assembling for departure.

There would be three members of the Ebola treatment team going in our convoy to Fish Town: Jonathan, an ER nurse from Montana, Henry, a sanitation expert from Uganda, and me. Two Liberian cooks, a supply specialist, a local guide, and a Liberian engineer would accompany us. We would have two pickup trucks and a Land Rover.

But before we could depart there was much work to be done. Two 55- gallon barrels of diesel fuel had to be unloaded and placed next to the generator that supplied power to the office. Then more diesel barrels had to be filled and placed securely in the bed of each pickup. There was also a stove, a safe, and boxes full of PPE uniforms, masks, gloves, chlorine, our personal suitcases, and a full propane tank. Naturally, the propane tank was secured next to a full diesel barrel. The truck was a rolling bomb that would be destroyed on sight in Iraq or Afghanistan. We designated it the smoking section.

Foam mattresses were secured on top of the Land Rover. These would be our future beds in Fish Town. They were about 4 inches thick and labeled "Supreme", indicating false advertising and future back problems.

The medical team stood around watching all the workers loading the supplies into the pickups. Jonathan decided to help with unloading the full diesel barrels and was rewarded with a crushed fingertip after it was pinned between a barrel and a concrete wall. I watched from the sidelines, supplying encouragement and medical care to the wounded.

Finally, about 1 pm, the trucks and Land Rover were packed, and we climbed aboard to begin our journey to Fish Town. We would travel the same hellish road we took to Bong County last week and then continue on for another 250 miles beyond. It would take us two days to travel 350 miles. I convinced myself that the roads could surely not get any worse past Bong County. I am a total fool.

The drive to Bong County was fairly uneventful with no dead bodies on the road, and we passed the Ebola Treatment Unit there in about 4 hours. The road, which was initially composed of irregular, broken asphalt, now gave way to compacted red dirt with more ruts and potholes than flat areas. The vehicles left a plume of red dust that often obscured the driver's vision to the point that we had to stop and wait for the dust to clear at times.

I rode in one of the pickups with a cook, Reginal, our supply specialist, Karmoh, and our driver, Alfred. We were supposed to stay together as a convoy, but Alfred was young and wanted to drive faster than the other vehicles.

I had to repeatedly ask him to slow down.

We arrived at Ganga City right at dusk and checked into the Alvino Hotel, the finest in town. There were 11 of us, 2 women and 9 men. There were five rooms available. Each tiny room had one double bed, and there were no rollaway beds. Since it was only for one night, we decided we could double up in the rooms. There was still one extra person, and I volunteered to share a room with the two young, pretty Liberian cooks. Unfortunately, my generous offer was declined, particularly so by the cooks, and one of the drivers went to find a room in another hotel. Jonathan and I decided to double up since we were the only two white guys and were aware of our strengths (beer drinking) and short comings (snoring).

The rooms had AC, cable TV, and self-flushing toilets. You are no doubt thinking self-flushing toilets are the high tech ones you see in airport restrooms that sense when a person is done and flushes automatically. I am talking about a whole other level of self-flushing toilets here.

In Liberia, self-flushing means doing your business, scooping buckets of water out of a giant barrel located in the bathroom, and then pouring the water down the toilet to force the contents down the sewer pipe. The water should be poured forcefully but not too forcefully because there might be a splash over accident that could be quite nasty. It is an interactive event that quickly brings humility.

I went down to the hotel restaurant to order some food. There was an extensive menu listing chicken, beef, hamburgers, shrimp, and fish as available options. I tried to order multiple listed items but was told they were out of everything except the fish. So I ordered the fish, grabbed a beer, and waited outside for my food.

After about 30 minutes there was still no food. Jonathan strolled up and reported that most of the team was going to another restaurant that had more food choices. I went inside and informed the waitress that I had decided to cancel my order and go elsewhere.

We walked to a nearby restaurant and reviewed the menu. Once again they were out of everything except chicken and rice, so we all ordered that. After eating, Jonathan and I headed back to the hotel since we were exhausted from the day's drive. Several of the younger men wanted to go out to a bar, so we parted ways.

Jonathan and I returned to the hotel, lowered the thermostat to the lowest possible setting, and climbed into bed. At 11:30 pm there was a knock on our door. The fish I ordered 4 hours ago was now ready. I replied that I had canceled the order and did not want the fish. The hotel clerk protested, but I said goodnight and shut the door.

The next morning we woke at 6 am to get ready for a long day of travel. The clerk reappeared and wanted me to pay for the fish I ordered last night. I told him if he still had the fish in the refrigerator, I would take it and pay for it. He did not return. There was some talk of sitting down for breakfast, but I persuaded the drivers to just go by a service station, grab some drinks and snacks, and hit the road.

Soon we were rolling down the "highway", which was really a glorified dirt road riddled with potholes and ruts. We were riding bucking broncos for the next several hours.

The young cook in my truck, Reginal, was unusually quiet this am and appeared tired. She was in the backseat and was able to nap through all this. Suddenly, about two hours into the drive, she sat bolt upright, rolled down the window, and vomited. We pulled over and let her finish on the side of the road. I gave her some water and toilet paper to clean her throat and face. I also gave her some Meclizine to chew and swallow to try and help her motion sickness. I advised her to sit up and look out at the horizon.

Reginal seemed to recover, and we started down the road again. I looked back to check on her, and she was texting and reading her cell phone messages. I warned her to not do that. I looked back again in a few minutes, and she had resumed her cell phone use. Twenty minutes later she threw open her truck door and vomited again. We stopped the truck once more and let her sit for a while.

I consulted with Jonathan, and he stated that maybe she was hung over from last night. I was surprised by this information since I had seen her at the restaurant the night before, and she had not been drinking. It turned out that after we left, two of the drivers had convinced the cooks to go with them to a nearby bar. I asked one of the drivers what the cooks had to drink. His reply, "Everything."

Armed with this new information, I gave her some Tylenol, Zantac, and another Meclizine. We continued down the road for another hour, and she seemed to be improving. We stopped to contain a leaking diesel barrel in one of the trucks (the one next to the propane tank, naturally). We secured the loose fill tops on the barrel and moved the luggage around so it would not get soaked in fuel.

The other cook and drivers brought food to Reginal to eat while we were waiting for the barrel repair. I saw this and walked over to warn her against putting solid food into an already upset stomach. I went back to help with the fuel leak, looked back, and saw her eating the fruit and crackers.

Twenty minutes down the road, we pulled over again for more vomiting, this time with partially digested food in the vomitus. This continued hourly until we stopped for a late lunch at 2:45 p.m. We gave Reginal a 45-minute rest break in the back of the Land Rover while we ate. I brought her a Sprite to drink, telling her to sip it slowly to see if she could keep it down. We had to get back on the road because it would be getting dark soon, and we still had several hours of driving to go. Reginal seemed better for a while, but after another hour of bouncing around in the truck, she started up again. It is a fate worse than death to be hung over, sick, and vomiting on a Liberian road.

We continued on our journey to Fish Town. Along the way, we passed through an Ebola checkpoint where we washed our hands in chlorinated water and had our temperatures taken. I counseled Reginal to try and not vomit since nausea and vomiting are early signs of Ebola. She made it through just fine, but Jonathan and the other cook were found to have low- grade temperatures by the inaccurate skin thermometers they use at such checkpoints. I had a moment of terror that we would be stuck here for days awaiting clearance. Jonathan and the cook drank some cool water and wiped their foreheads with a wet cloth. After 5 minutes they passed (< 38 degrees Centigrade), and we were allowed to continue on.

We stopped at a church in a small village on one of our frequent stops. The young children were intrigued by me and watched me intently. I was wearing a Daniel Johnson T-shirt that says, "Hi how are you" with a frog-like drawing. I remarked to Jonathan that they must think I am a cartoon character, like Mickey Mouse. He corrected me replying, "Not Mickey, more like Goofy."

I approached a small group of children, and one of them ran away from me. I held my hand out to the others, and finally a brave child stepped up and touched me. After that it became a dare among the children to touch me. I don't know if they had seen a white man before, but if so, not many.

As we drove along, the terrain changed from a few trees and rolling hills to frank jungle where you could not walk five feet off the road due to the dense foliage. The road narrowed to one lane, and the trees and vines seemed to reach out and grab at our vehicles as we drove along. There were abandoned, rusting vehicles on the sides of the road that were slowly being swallowed up by the encroaching jungle. At nightfall, we finally pulled up to the Best 8 Guest House on the outskirts of Fish Town where many of our team would be staying the next few weeks.

It had been a long two days of travel, and I was relieved that we had arrived safely. I was the first doctor in our team to arrive in Fish Town, and I felt the weight of responsibility on me. I had been passing out lots of Tylenol to many of my team members for minor aches and pains.

Reginal had recovered and thanked me for my medications and attention.

We have much work ahead of us with evaluating our future ETU, meeting with local leaders, engineers, and healthcare providers, and communicating our findings back to Monrovia and Minneapolis.

Here we go.

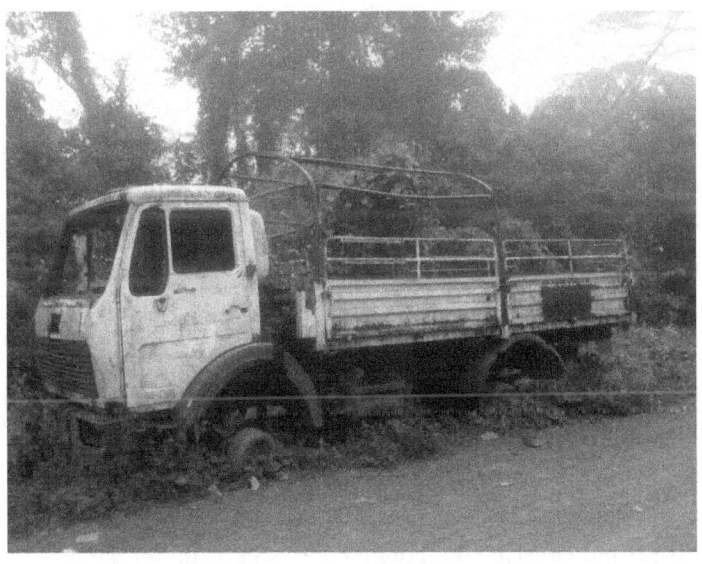

Abandoned vehicle on side of national highway

Fish Town, River Gee, Liberia

Dear Family and Friends,

Fish Town has no fish. It did have fish in the rivers and ponds when initially settled, but all the fish were seined out. There are plans for a restocking program in the future, but for right now the only fish come from neighboring counties and a coastal town, Harper, a four-hour drive away.

We are staying at the Best 8 Guest House two miles out of Fish Town proper. There is a generator to supply electricity, but it is totally unreliable and often cuts out at night, leaving us without fans to blow the warm humid air over our sweating bodies. Our rooms are like caves with expertly designed windows that do not allow sunlight or breezes to invade.

There is no running water. We bathe out of buckets filled with brownish river water. There are self-flushing toilets that I have previously described. There is no sink. You brush your teeth over the toilet bowl and spit. There is no on-site bar or restaurant. The kitchen area is located outside and consists of an open charcoal grill under a palm leaf covered open-air structure. There is a freezer, but since the generator only runs intermittently, your drinks may be either frozen or warm. It goes without saying that there is no Internet. In my room there are complimentary condoms placed on the bed stand. This is a first class establishment.

We sit out in the dirt parking lot whenever possible to eat, drink, and talk. They bring a table out for us most of the time. We socialize while chickens stroll around us. There is a road side stand right next to us that sells fruits and vegetables and blares out music from sunup to sundown. We have dubbed this the Worst 8 Motel.

Fish Town has a population of about 3,500 people. There is the usual dusty, potholed road down the center of town. There is a restaurant we frequent that we have named the Waffle House. I don't think it even serves waffles, but it does have eggs and pancakes. The only meal I ever had there was spaghetti with Spam. It tasted just like it sounds. Terry, our Texas engineer, loves this spot for breakfast, so this has become a rendezvous point in the morning.

There is another restaurant that I prefer called Domeny's. It sits on top of a hill and has a patio, a bar, a good breeze, and a commanding view of the surrounding jungle. There is usually loud Afro/Pop/Reggae/Rap music blasting from the inside. Occasionally, a local dancer will appear to entertain us. His name is Sammy, and he has more dance moves than Michael Jackson ever did. The actual spelling of the dining establishment is "Rastuarant", so we have nicknamed it as such. It is our gathering site in case of an emergency evacuation. At least it has beer.

I have been making the city rounds meeting and making nice with the local health authorities, mayor, and engineers. If our ETU is to get a good start, we will need the support of the local leaders and community. Much of the business in Fish Town is conducted in bars, so I am well trained for that. I think they like me because I always make a point to say we are here to assist the Liberian people and not give orders or take control of the Ebola emergency response. And, of course, I always buy them a beer.

In the three days I have been here, I have toured our future ETU every day. I have toured it with the construction foreman and local politicians. I have toured it with the German owned construction crew that is building it, and I have toured it with the medical personnel from the U.S Department of Defense.

There are several minor design flaws in the ETU layout that we will need to modify to ensure patient, visitor, and employee safety. So far every group I have met has been cooperative and has demonstrated willingness to solve problems for the good of Ebola patients and the community.

The German construction representatives had, paradoxically, no Germans among them. The project manager was from Denmark, and the chief engineer was from the Philippines. Our ETU layout is unique due to its hillside location. The original layout has been drastically altered since filtering down through the multiple layers of Liberian bureaucracy and Ebola emergency response organizations. The Denmark project manager looked the final layout over and proclaimed, "This is what happens when you get doctors involved!" I countered with, "I hope you don't get sick."

A dozen U.S. Army medical and support personnel arrived on a Black Hawk helicopter the other day. A Lt. Colonel physician who is an Infectious Disease specialist led them. I toured the ETU with him and answered his questions. The Army is in Fish Town to set up hot and cold training for Liberians that will be working in our ETU. We discussed the changes that needed to be made in the ETU layout from a medical point of view. He was supportive of the changes we had proposed and even invited our physicians and nurses to participate in the upcoming ETU training classes. The Army medical group also toured both the old and new high schools for possible cold training sites. Only one had toilets, if you call a closet with a hole in the concrete floor a toilet.

The last stop the Army made was to look at a possible housing site for their upcoming stay here in one week. It is owned by a local official who accompanied them during their brief visit to Fish Town. It is called the County Guest House and has a total of seven rooms. The Army had originally been promised all of the rooms in advance, but when they visited yesterday they were told only five rooms would be available. One of the officers asked whom they could speak with to get the other two rooms. The local official answered, "Me." Sometimes, even the U.S. Army doesn't get its way.

I have kept busy writing and sending reports back to Monrovia and Minneapolis about our activities and interactions with local leaders here in Fish Town. Internet access has been obtained through a local official who allows me to sit in his lobby. It is glacially slow, but it is better than nothing.

Our future employee housing is several miles away from the ETU and is still under construction. Hopefully, it will be available for occupancy before Christmas. We are still waiting for the tents to arrive, a well for water needs to be drilled, and a septic tank needs to be finished. All of us staying at the Worst 8 Motel are actually looking forward to moving into tents.

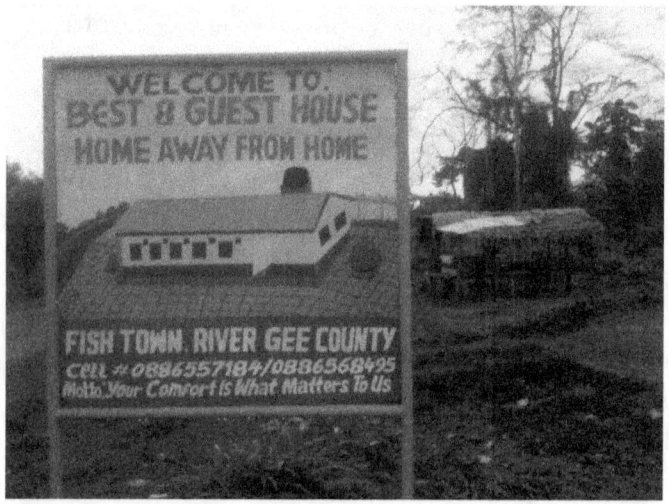

The Worst 8 Motel

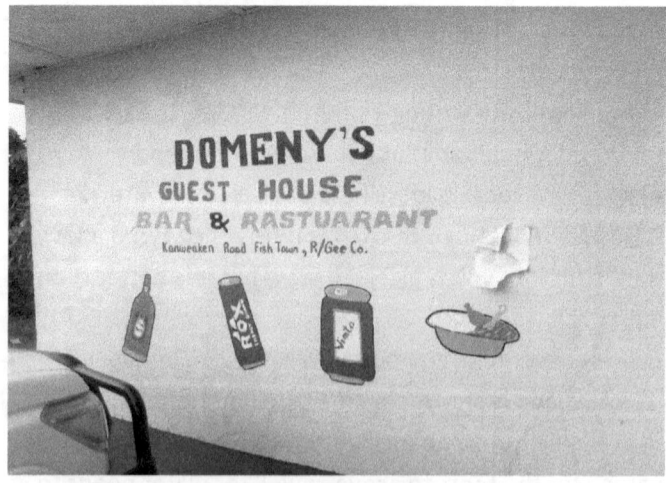

Domeny's Rastuarant

Ebola Rumor Detectives

Dear Family and Friends,

Since arriving in Fish Town, there have been occasional reports of possible Ebola patients in the surrounding villages. We gather as much information as possible from hospitals, clinics, and citizens and then try to confirm or discredit the stories. The cell phone coverage here is extremely poor, and many villages have none. In some of the villages, the few cell phones are hung in trees at the center of the village in case a connection is made and a call received. It may take hours or days for an Ebola report to be confirmed or discounted.

The first rumor we investigated was that of a woman who was admitted to an outside clinic with the complaint of diarrhea for several weeks. Jonathan and Kelsy rode out on motorcycles to the outlying clinic to get more information. After an hour ride they were able to meet with the Liberian nurse stationed there. From talking with the nurse they discovered that the patient had been experiencing diarrhea for years, and it was made worse by milk ingestion. Yes doctors, she had lactose intolerance. Case closed.

The second rumor was more serious. A woman had first arrived at a nearby hospital and was then referred to a temporary "mini-ETU" that was operational and run by Samaritan's Purse, another health care group. The patient complained of vomiting, diarrhea, and possible fever for three days. She denied contact with a sick person or dead body.

She was brought into the triage booth to be further evaluated with temperature and additional history. The medical personnel in their full PPE outfits frightened her, and she refused to go in to have an Ebola blood test done. She called her husband, and he came and picked her up. They told the health care workers that they were going to travel to another hospital, but they never showed up there. After a several day hunt, the woman was finally tracked down, but she was no longer feeling ill. She probably had one of the dozen other causes for diarrhea and fever that exist in Liberia.

There have been no confirmed cases of Ebola in our county, River Gee, in the past month. We are on the eastern fringe of Liberia, and most of the ongoing Ebola cases have been around Monrovia, Bong County, and areas close to Sierra Leone. Even those areas have been reporting a decreasing number of Ebola cases. I will take this as a blessing to the Liberian people, but I had anticipated a more active role in the Ebola epidemic.

The Fish Town ETU is making slow progress towards becoming a reality. Almost all of the structures are up, and they are putting in the plumbing and electricity. Heavy afternoon thunderstorms and torrential rains the past few days have slowed the construction. We had hoped to be open by December 21st, but it is now looking more like January 1st or later. We are looking forward to opening it whether there are Ebola patients or not.

The rest of our medical team arrived this week. There is a shortage of housing in Fish Town, and some members of our team are sleeping on foam mattresses in hotel lobbies.

Our employee camp, nicknamed the Fish Tank, is also behind schedule. An afternoon rainstorm caused a concrete block wall in the septic tank to collapse, and it will need to be rebuilt. When completed, it should be great with 24- hour electricity, running water, cold-water showers, and toilets that actually flush with just a touch of a handle!

The Department of Defense is returning after Christmas and will begin hot and cold training for our employees who have not yet had this training. Many of the doctors and nurses are looking forward to working with the Army. It will be a good refresher course in the donning and doffing of PPE and the Ebola treatment protocols.

Love,

Joe

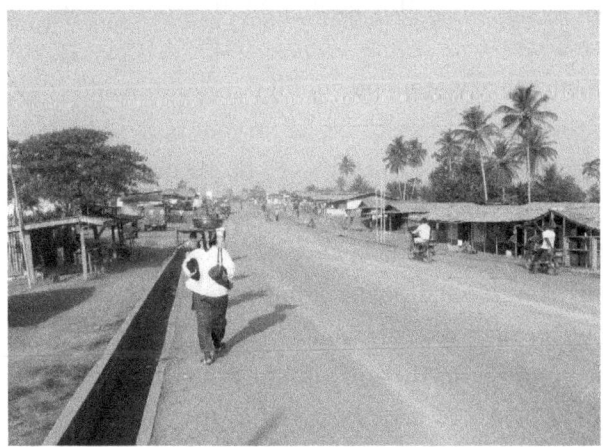

Main Street Fish Town, Liberia

How to Take a Bucket Bath in Liberia

In response to no inquiries, I will tell you the best way to take a bath out of a bucket in Liberia. Get up in the morning before the generator shuts off around 6:30 am so you can see around your room. Get dressed and attack your top objective of the day, be it touring the unfinished ETU unit, running down Ebola rumors, meeting local officials, or grocery shopping. About 2 or 3 pm you are soaked with sweat, covered with dust, and wish you had never come here. You then go out to the pump well and fill a couple of buckets with brownish river water to take to your room. If you are not already drenched in sweat, you will be after pumping the water. Once in your bathroom, you strip down to your birthday suit and step into a tiled shower with teasing plumbing fixtures protruding from the walls that do not produce water.

Take a bucket of water and pour it over your head. Enjoy the cool water as it cascades down your body, grab the shampoo and get your hair lathered up. After that it is time for the bar of soap to reach those expanses and crevices of your body that make life great. Now grab the other bucket of water and slowly pour it over your head letting the water rinse off the shampoo and soap. An extra bucket of water for good measure is always a nice finish. Step out of the tiled area and dry off. Enjoy the coolness and cleanliness that soothes your body.

This is the highlight of your day. It will last for about 30 minutes.

Ebola Response Team Conversation

Occasionally, when sitting around in the morning or evening, the conversation will eventually turn to important topics such as bowel movements. Individuals will freely offer detailed information on the current state of their bowels. Those eating street food will usually report diarrhea or "running stomach" as they say in Liberia. Other individuals complain about constipation due to the large amount of rice in their diet.

Being doctors and nurses we offer medical advice to each other. The people with constipation should eat more street food. The people with diarrhea should eat more rice and less street food.

I usually try to stay out of such table talk because I have listened to stories about patients' bowels for 30 years. While it is of infinite importance to little old ladies and gastroenterology doctors, I couldn't give a sh*t.

Other topics covered include insect stings and bites, bruises and abrasions, and how miserable your night of non-sleep was. There are few mosquitoes where we are staying, but there are still plenty of wasps, biting ants, and horseflies to keep you on guard at all times.

If a Nairobi fly crawls on you, you must be careful to flick it off. Smashing it or rubbing it against your skin will bring instant severe burning pain from the chemical toxin it carries in its body. The burn will eventually blister, and a wide swath of your skin will peel off. The pain will last for two weeks. It is a most unpleasant experience that I would like to avoid.

The bruises and abrasions are sustained during normal daily activities such as climbing in and out of pickups and Land Rovers, jumping across ditches, and bumping into furniture in the darkness of your room. I have applied many Band-Aids and triple antibiotic ointment to the wounded in our group. I carry the Band-Aids and ointment in my backpack at all times along with a bottle of Tylenol.

It has become a competition now to quantify the abject misery experienced by an individual during the night. Laying on your caved in foam mattress and sweating with a fan blowing warm humid air on you will get you no points. That is a given. There must be a stinging or biting insect involved, loud music or roosters crowing outside your window at 6 am, or nighttime trauma suffered to get you in the game. A combination of all three would be a hat trick.

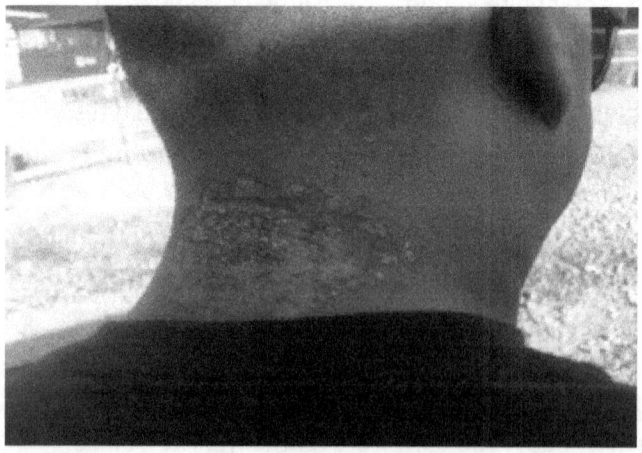

Nairobi Fly aftermath

Fish Town Market Day

Dear Family and Friends,

Thursday is the big weekly outdoor market day in Fish Town, and since I had no meetings to attend today, I decided to go grocery shopping with our cooks, Reginal and Jebbeh. Reginal has taken a shine to me since I cared for her during the tortuous, bilious ride to Fish Town. We have been eating nothing but chicken and Spam since our arrival here, and I am hungry for fish and beef.

The market is located on the main road just outside of town and was packed with vendors and shoppers when we arrived at 9:30 am. There was the usual assortment of chicken feet, hot peppers, bananas, papayas, and eggplant.

There were no tomatoes, cucumbers, or cabbage available. We located the fresh fish area at the back of the market and examined the offerings. There were many small fish such as perch and mackerel for sale, but we finally found a seller with some red snapper.

The fish were not nearly as big as the ones we had in Monrovia, but they looked fresh, so we bought six fish for $10. We also purchased some onions and potatoes. We asked about "cow meat", which is what beef is called around here, and were told there is a town about 20 miles away that might have some.

We climbed into the truck with Alfred and started the journey. We traveled the usual rutted dirt road, but I appreciated the surrounding hills and valleys a bit more when rested. As we passed through the small villages, the cooks rolled down the windows and asked the pedestrians where they could find some cow meat. Most did not know, but finally a person named a certain village with a butcher shop. After 45 minutes we arrived at the village, parked the truck, and got out on foot.

The first few food venders knew nothing about cow meat, but we eventually found a young boy who seemed to know where we could find some. We followed him along the main street and he started to lead us down an alleyway. Reginal asked me to stay on the main street while she and the other cook checked it out. I have never felt in danger here, but I heeded her advice and stayed on the main street. A few minutes later Reginal reappeared and motioned me across the street.

We walked inside an open wooden structure with dogs snoozing on the floor and cow carcasses hanging from ceiling hooks. The intestines were lying on a table, no doubt being saved for some Liberian delicacy. The meat looked and smelled fresh, so we bought ten pounds of steak for $40. At $4/pound I considered that a good buy.

I observed that the main butcher had his left forearm in a sling and noted visible swelling when I peered through an opening. He stated he had a bad fall three days ago, landing on his outstretched left palm. He went to a local health clinic and was told he had a fracture and was given a sling. No x-ray was done or splint applied. I identified myself as a doctor and asked if I might examine his arm.

His left forearm was swollen to about twice normal size with tenderness to palpation just proximal to his wrist.

There were some superficial scratches overlying but no erythema or warmth. He was able to move his fingers and thumb well and denied sensory loss. He stated it was getting better and he was told to wear the sling for several more weeks. I had no doubt he had broken both his distal radius and ulna. Such is the medical care of fractures in rural Liberia.

We made the return trip to Fish Town and purchased some cooking oil, canned vegetables, rice, spices, and black pepper. I treated the cooks and driver to soft drinks, and they dropped me off at my hotel. We are going to have the red snapper tonight and the steaks tomorrow night. Let the feasting begin.

There is talk of a road trip to Harper on Sunday. Harper is a coastal town and receives regular shipments of products and food from other towns and countries by boat. There is also a high probability of finding shrimp and fresh produce, such as tomatoes, cabbage, cucumbers, apples, and oranges. Just thinking about it makes my mouth water. There are plenty of bananas, papayas, and coconuts here, but if I eat any more I will start swinging from the trees.

Love,

Joe

Liberia Election Day

December 20, 2014

There is a major election coming up this Saturday. Much like the United States, each county (state) elects two senators to represent them on a national level in Monrovia. They are elected for 9-year terms that are staggered. River Gee has no less than nine candidates running for office this year. Whoever gets the most votes wins. There is no runoff unless the top two candidates tie.

The other day there was a debate among the candidates at city hall. The building was packed, and people spilled out of the entranceway and crowded around the windows to listen. Many people were wearing T-shirts proclaiming their allegiance to a certain candidate. Vans and trucks covered with political banners slowly drove the streets filled with passengers shouting out support for their candidate.

I have listened to some of the candidates on the radio, and much of the debate circles around jobs and Ebola. There is an 85% unemployment rate throughout the country. Most families get by on an income of two to four dollars a day. 85% of the population is under the International poverty level.

In Fish Town there are currently hundreds of workers employed to help build the Ebola treatment unit and our future camp. Every day I see dozens of men standing outside the two sites asking for jobs. There are makeshift stands set up outside each site to sell food and water to the workers. Although Ebola has taken many lives in Liberia, it has also provided a wealth of jobs for its citizens.

We have been warned to stay away from downtown and crowds on election day. UN armored vehicles will be patrolling the streets with machine guns mounted on their roofs. Liberia has just ended a brutal and bloody civil war a little over ten years ago, and the democratic process is still young and fragile.

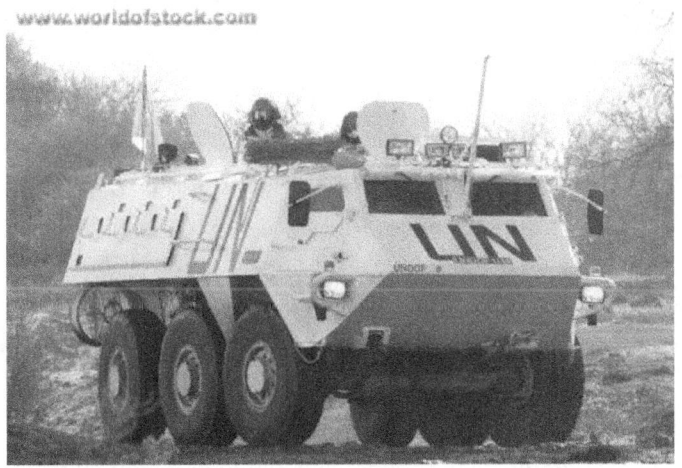

Road Trip To Harper

We have been in Fish Town for only a week and have already grown tired of the dusty stores, restaurants, and bars. There is a coastal town, Harper, only a short four-hour drive away. It promises beautiful beaches, fresh seafood, and beachside resorts with air conditioning, plumbing, electricity, and Internet. It is the Shangri-La of our miserable existence here in Fish Town.

Nothing much ever gets done on Sundays in Fish Town, so it was chosen as the best day to go. An elite crew was selected: our driver, Alfred, who likes to drive fast and play loud American music, our two cute, young cooks, Reginal and Jebbeh, our two WASH (Water, Sanitation, and Hygiene) specialists from Uganda, George and Henry, Kelsy, and me.

We traveled in a 4-wheel drive crew cab Ford F150 pickup since the Land Rover would be needed to pick up more members of our team coming from Monrovia. They would be arriving by UN helicopters, indicating extremely poor judgment and a sissy way to get here. Our team coordinator would be with them and would no doubt start scheduling senseless meetings to justify her position. It was the perfect time for a road trip.

Our expectations were high as we departed Fish Town. We left shortly after 8 am to beat the rush hour traffic (insert joke here). The road to Harper was not too bad by Liberian standards. There were brief stretches of road that were actually smooth dirt. Because there were seven of us, two rode in the bed of the pickup. Since I was the oldest and whitest, I volunteered to do so. Henry graciously volunteered to accompany me.

We passed through several villages along the way and even crossed the River Gee for which the county is named. We stopped to walk around, take pictures, and get a good look. River Gee is fast moving with rapids and waterfalls. I would not want to kayak or canoe it. The villages were made up of mud brick huts with thatched roofs, and there was usually a petrol station, bar, and restaurant.

Henry and I rode in the bed of the pickup and held on for dear life as Alfred negotiated the potholes and mud traps that characterize Liberian roads. Whenever a motorcycle or other vehicle went past us, we were engulfed by a plume of red dust. It was particularly bad when a large semitrailer was in front of us, and we were waiting to pass. Henry and I ducked down behind the cab of the truck at those times, but dust still got to us.

The geography changed to many high mountains and valleys covered with thick jungle foliage. It was decidedly the wildest looking area we have traveled through so far. The road narrowed to just a single track with occasional wide expanses where vehicles had previously swerved to avoid particularly deep mud holes or potholes.

We entered Harper, and my hopes and expectations soared when we suddenly found ourselves driving on intact, paved roads. Of course, this was short lived. Many buildings in downtown Harper were just the concrete skeletons of their previous lives after being burned or destroyed during the civil war a dozen years ago. These concrete remains were now empty or occupied by families with boards over the open windows and roofs. There were the usual wooden, tin roofed buildings that are ubiquitous to Liberia, but the once great town of Harper was no more.

We could see the ocean and palm fringed beach as we drove along, following the main road to where it ended on a cove. Everyone was tired, so we got out to stretch our legs and feel the sand and ocean. When I climbed out of the bed of the pickup, one of the cooks asked me, "Dr. Joe, why is your face red?" I immediately thought that I did not apply enough sunscreen that morning, but when I touched my face, there was red dirt on my finger. My whole body was covered with the red dust thrown up on our travel here. I walked down to the beach and washed my face and hands in the cool Atlantic water. The water was clean and the sand soft on my feet. It felt great.

There was a bar near the beach that was open, and we ordered cold sodas all around. We took our drinks and walked around the beach and rocks, soaking our feet, absorbing the beautiful views, and taking pictures of each other. We talked to the bar's owner and her son to get information about local restaurants, hotels, and grocery stores.

Alas, we picked the worst possible day of the week to visit. All the markets and restaurants are closed on Sunday. There was no seafood to buy or eat. In fact, there was no food to be had in all of Harper on this day. We did get two names of hotels in Harper, so we decided to check them out.

The first hotel was located downtown across from a burned out building and an intact church. We could hear the choir singing as we exited the truck. As we entered the lobby we noted the complimentary condom dispensary right next to the reservation desk. After calling out for several minutes, the manager appeared, and we told him we were looking for possible rooms for our group should we take a rest and relaxation leave from Fish Town. He gave us a tour of his fine establishment.

The rooms on the first floor were worse than our rooms in the Worst 8 Motel in Fish Town. There were sad looking twin beds that sagged in the middle, no room fans, and a shared bathroom of bare toilets without seats. The rooms cost $15 a night. They were the perfect rooms for committing suicide or overdosing on drugs.

The second floor rooms were initially promising with nice double beds, private bathrooms, and AC units mounted on the walls. These rooms cost $35 a night and were the top of the line for this establishment.

I inquired about the generators and was told they run from 7 p.m. to 7 a.m...not bad. I asked if the air conditioners worked. The manager replied that they were not connected to the generator because they cost too much money to run. "So you have them and don't use them?" I asked. "Exactly," he replied.

We moved on to the second hotel. It was on a beachfront several blocks away from the downtown area. The visible building was of new construction, definitely something built after the war. There was a large expanse of lush green grass in front with palm trees providing shade.

We parked on the grass and asked to see the owner. A man working in the yard pointed to a pair of individuals seated under the palm trees.

We walked over and met Mr. John Ballout. He was playing Scrabble with a woman and asked her to get up and bring some chairs for us. He was of Lebanese descent, as are many of the major grocery and hotel owners in Liberia. We introduced ourselves and told him we were looking for rooms to rent for episodic visits by members of our medical team. He nodded and said he had eight rooms total, but only five were available this week. We asked to see them, and he called a lady to give us a tour.

On the outside the hotel was not that impressive, but when we entered the main lobby, we knew we had found the Promised Land. The lobby was huge and expansive and furnished with soft looking sofas and chairs. The floors were made of beautiful white marble that was sparkling clean and flowed throughout the entire hotel. There was a big screen TV set up and a table with a tea service.

We went to see a room and were once again blown away. The bedroom was huge and filled with natural light. There was a king bed, fan, and satellite TV. The large, louvered windows looked out on the beach and ocean with a pleasant, cool breeze blowing in. The bathroom was oversized and had a sink, toilet, mirrors, and tub. You still had to flush your own toilet, but that was expected. Electricity was provided 24 hours a day, and they would cook meals for you at an additional cost.

The rooms cost $50/night, and I wanted to immediately move there. Unfortunately, we were on a fact-finding mission, and we had to return to Fish Town that night. I wrote down the names and phone numbers associated with the hotel to pass the information up the chain of command of our group.

We left Harper hungry and empty handed. We stopped at a large village 30 minutes out of town that seemed alive with activity, despite being a Sunday. We found some spaghetti noodles, beef Spam, tomato sauce, and fresh, warm bread for dinner. It was not the dinner I had hoped for, but they were the only items available.

We began the four-hour return journey to Fish Town. Kelsy and I rode in the bed of the pickup while the Liberians and Uganda folks rode in the cab. As we passed through the villages, I am sure we made a strange sight with the black people inside the cab and the white people riding in the back. Groups of young children enthusiastically waved at us as we passed through villages. We felt like we were in a Christmas parade and should have been throwing candy to them

We drove through one village at top speed and passed a bar full of Liberian men drinking beer and watching soccer. I toasted the men with a beer bottle in my hand as we passed and received an outburst of laughter and cheers. I am pretty sure I would have been instantly fired if the people in Minneapolis saw what I was doing.

We approached an impasse on the return trip. A minivan was stuck in a deep mud hole, and no one could pass on either side. Several men were attempting to push it out, only to receive a mud shower from the spinning tires. Another minivan tied a rope to the stuck vehicle and was finally able to pull it out. Naturally, the previously stuck minivan immediately attacked the mud hole again but miraculously cleared it this time. We followed immediately behind in our 4- wheel drive truck before any other vehicle could get stuck. We are decidedly badass.

We finally arrived in Fish Town right at dusk. Additional members of our medical team joined us, and there were toasts and greetings all around. We were glad to be back together, but there was still much work to be done before we could move into our ETU and Fish Tank together.

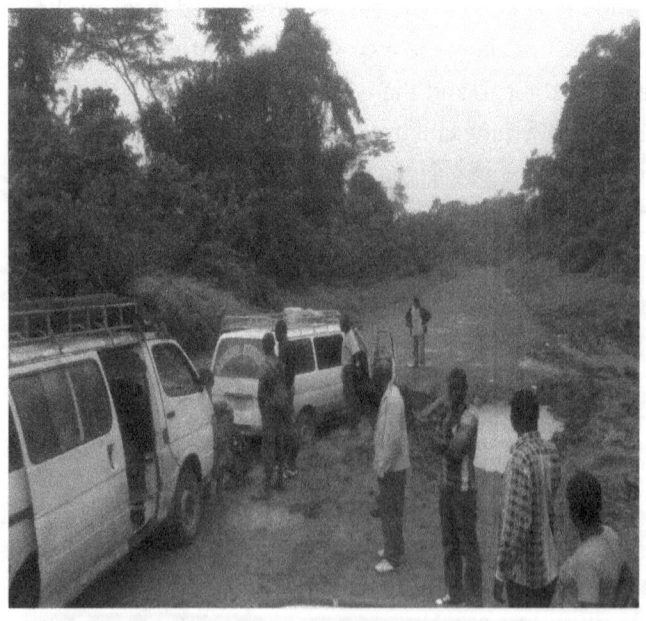

Stuck in the mud on the national highway in Liberia

Merry Christmas from Fish Town, Liberia

Dear Family and Friends,

There is a family that lives next to our hotel parking lot. There are eight children, two girls and six boys. They are all under 12 years of age. Their father is building a house for the family back off the road. At the present time it is just a bare timber skeleton, and he works on it daily. They are currently living in a small thatch-roofed mud brick house with a charcoal grill to cook on. I occasionally buy papayas and pineapples that they offer for sale. They only cost 25 to 50 cents apiece.

I sit outside in the morning and evening and watch them play. I have noticed that all the children wear the same dirty T-shirts and pants every day. The mother's name is Josephina. The youngest child is usually strapped to her back.

I have decided to adopt them as my Christmas family this year. I can buy them gently used shirts and trousers for two to three dollars apiece at the local market. When does $40 ever get a chance to bring a little happiness to an entire family?

Merry Christmas everyone.

Love,

Joe

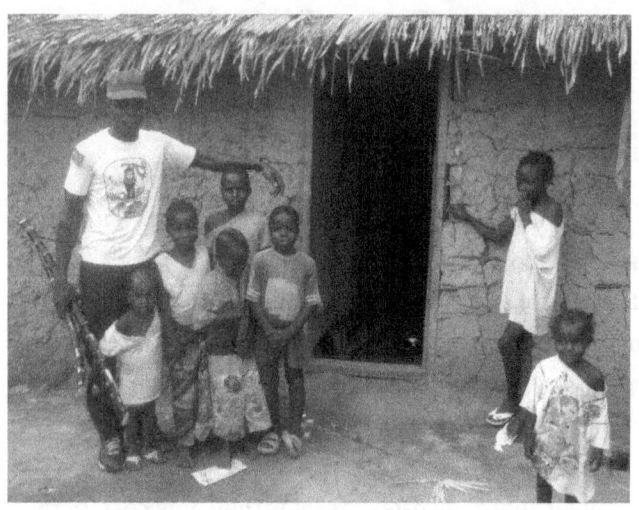

Family I adopted for Christmas

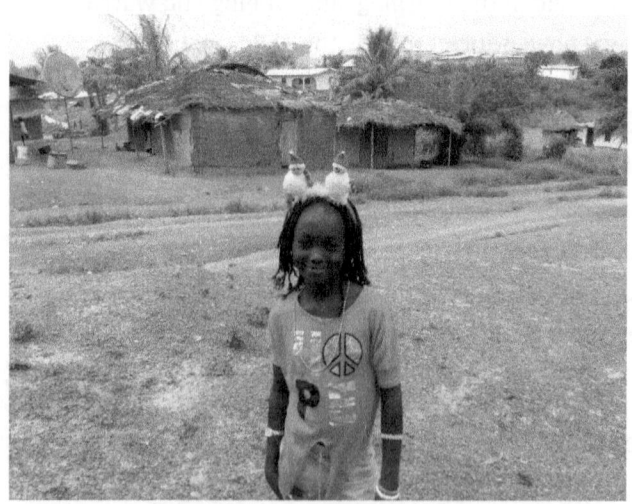

Christmas Day in Fish Town

Christmas Eve and Christmas Day 2014

Fish Town, Liberia

Dear Family and Friends,

It is Christmas Eve, and my first priority this morning is to go to Philip's office. Philip is a local administrator for the German construction company that is building our ETU. He has the most reliable Internet connection in Fish Town and has been kind enough to allow us to sit in his main lobby and use it. We try to stay out of the way, but it is a small room, and all our electrical cords stretch across the main passageway. He patiently steps over the cords and maneuvers his way around the bodies.

We have decided to give him a Christmas present as a way to thank him for allowing us to use his office and Internet. I have seen and met with him several times at Cece's, the local hang bar. I bought him four bottles of his favorite beer, Guinness, and a bottle of an Argentina Malbec that I hope is good. I also wrote a combination thank you note and Christmas card on a folded yellow legal page and placed it next to the plastic bag containing the beverages.

That evening I received a knock on my door. It was one of the motel workers with a manila envelope addressed to our medical team and me. I opened it and found a neatly typed letter from Philip thanking us for the beer and wine. He was away from his family this Christmas and understood how hard it was to be away from home this time of year.

He was glad to have us as partners and friends in Fish Town. It was elegantly signed and dated. It was the only Christmas card I received this year.

Later on that evening, my teammates and I sat outside and shared a bottle of wine and a few beers. Kelsy brought some Christmas decorations, and we put them up over the entrance to the motel. That night I dreamt of what Santa Claus would bring me. I hope it is a Learjet so I can get out of this place.

Christmas morning I awoke and opened my bedroom door to discover…a Learjet! No, of course not, but there was a small amount of candy wrapped in a colorful napkin hanging from my outside doorknob. I was not the only recipient, as all of our team at the motel received one. There was even a small piece of chocolate that is extremely hard to find around here.

I sat outside in the coolness of the morning and enjoyed the silence. The mother of the family I adopted appeared with a large bowl of three ripe papayas. She gave them to me as a Christmas gift. I also noted that she was wearing the yellow shirt with spiders detailed on it that I had purchased for one of her sons. I guess she decided to keep it for herself. My Christmas spirit took one step backwards.

Other team members gradually joined me at the breakfast table we set up outside. Not only was it Christmas Day, but it was also Henry's birthday! Henry is deathly afraid of snakes and hates my Snake Farm shirt. Coincidentally, that morning the pineapple farmer across the road called out to us that there was a snake in his driveway. Naturally, I immediately rushed over to investigate the first snake sighting.

Sure enough, there was a small pit viper about 2 feet in length writhing around on the ground with a frog in its mouth. The farmer had already delivered a mortal wound to the snake with a stick. As we walked up, the frog escaped from the snake's mouth and hopped away. I took a few pictures as the snake expired.

Henry appeared late for breakfast, and we sang "Happy Birthday" to him. A few chocolate bars were given to him as a gift. I mentioned to him about the snake across the road, and he recoiled. After I reassured him a dozen times that the snake was dead, he agreed to go look at it. He stood 10 feet away from the snake and glared at it. We returned to the breakfast table to continue the birthday celebration. It was the perfect set-up for my birthday surprise to Henry.

I briefly returned to my room to retrieve the rubber snake that my good friend Steve gave me for security from would be thieves. So far it had been 100% effective. I put the rubber snake in my shorts' front pocket (insert trouser snake joke here) and inconspicuously returned to the table. Henry was casually soaking his tea bag when I pulled the rubber snake out and pretended to be fighting it. Henry jumped up and ran across the parking area screaming. Everyone at the table fell over laughing except, of course, Henry. He refused to return to the breakfast table until the rubber snake was removed. Happy birthday Henry! I love you. Mission accomplished.

Christmas morning brought not only papayas and snakes, but also a passing trailer rumbling by with large wooden boxes on it labeled ARC. Our tents had finally arrived!   Terry, our Texas engineer, swung by in a Land Rover looking for help unloading the newly arrived trailer. We all saddled up and climbed aboard. When we arrived at our future camp, there were already a dozen laborers present. I evaluated the size and weight of the wooden boxes and decided that I should step aside and let the younger men do the unloading.

I offered enthusiastic verbal support to the workers and once again administered first aid to the wounded. Two workers sustained small cuts on their fingers that I cleansed with purified water and applied antibiotic ointment and Band-Aids to. It was definitely low- tech medicine, but it was something. I loaned a pair of work gloves to a worker, and they disappeared. I am a slow learner.

Terry led the workers as they attempted to erect the tents. The US Army tents, of course, came with unintelligible instructions and diagrams that were undecipherable. After three hours of futile effort, Terry and the workers gave up and went to lunch.

I caught a ride to the Waffle House and had an egg sandwich. Afterwards, Kelsy and I walked to a nearby Lutheran church I had visited earlier. I was told there would be a special Christmas service at 1 p.m., but when we arrived, there was no one in the church. We were surrounded by several groups of children who apparently thought we were Santa Claus.

I caught a ride back to town, bought some beer at Cece's, and headed home. It was time for a bucket bath and a beer. Tonight, I will call home at 5 p.m. and talk to my wife, June, and my daughter, Ellen, for a long time. Our medical team will have a group dinner tonight with fresh fish, cow meat, rice, and pineapple. It will be a delicious feast.

It is not the best Christmas I have ever had, but it is far from the worst. Last year at this time my mother lay dying in my living room under hospice care. Your life is all about perspective. Make it a positive one.

Love,

Joe

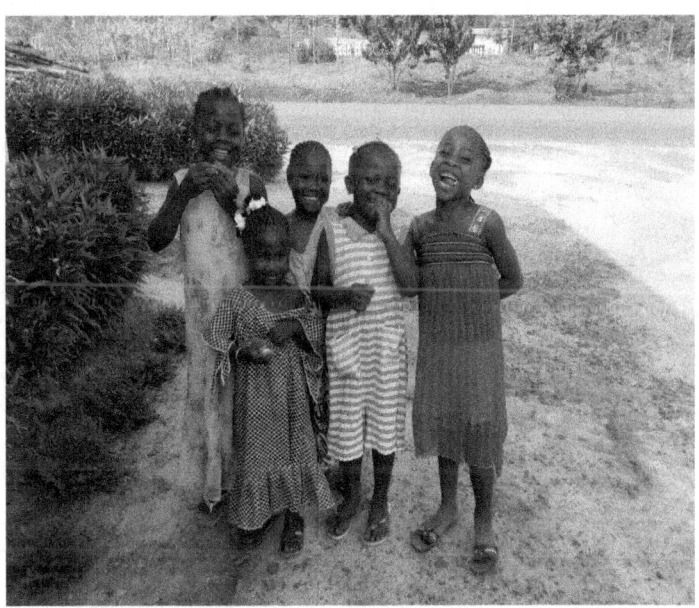

Liberian sisters on Christmas Day

The US Army Arrives for
ETU Training

Today the army arrived to lead their ETU training course for local Fish Town residents hoping to work in our ETU. Our medical team was invited to attend and even participate in the training exercises. See one, do one, teach one. They arrived by Chinook helicopters, and we met them at the landing site. I had never seen a Chinook helicopter and was excited about doing so. A group of us drove out to the helicopter landing site just outside of town and waited.

While waiting, I remembered a scene from the movie *Forrest Gump* where Forrest and Bubba are being flown by helicopter into Vietnam to begin their combat duty. "Fortunate Son'" by Creedence Clearwater Revival is blasting in the background. I have the song on my iPad and played it for our small group. It is the only helicopter song I know.

We sat in the shade on crudely made but functional wooden benches. Barely audible at first, but more of a vibration in the air, we heard the low thumping sounds...the helicopters are coming!

I raced out to the landing pad with my camera. The thumping sounds grew louder, and soon one and then the other Chinook helicopter cleared the tree line. Chinook helicopters have not one, but two large propellers and can carry much heavier loads than standard Army helicopters. One helicopter overshot the landing pad and had to turn around. The other one honed right in and slowly floated to the ground. I was standing about 100 feet away from the landing site and would now receive a painful lesson about helicopters.

Rotor wash! The helicopter blades created a veritable tornado of wind and dust that enveloped me and everyone else within 50 yards. I fled to the cover of our Land Rover. The second helicopter approached and flew low over a nearby house. As it passed over, the tin roof of the house was lifted off and thrown to the side. The locals and I raced over to the house to see if anyone was injured. Fortunately, no one was in the house at the time, and no one was hurt.

After the helicopter landed, a large ramp in the back opened up and armed soldiers dispersed around the site to provide security. The rest of the troops followed, and they started unloading boxes of supplies. A group of three officers checked out the damage at the neighboring house. I was told a report will be filed, damages assessed, Army attorneys involved, and the roof would be replaced. It may take weeks for all this to play out.

I approached a couple of men who appeared to be in charge. I met Captain Daniel, a family practice physician from Tennessee. He will lead the ETU training here. We spoke briefly and agreed to meet later that day for a tour of Fish Town. On the way home I drove the Land Rover myself. It was a powerful feeling to be driving a monster vehicle on a Liberian road. My testosterone level jumped at least 100 points.

I returned at 3 p.m. to meet Captain Daniel and the nurse manager, Mark. We first drove to the Fish Town government run medical clinic to see if the Army PPE uniforms had arrived. We were ushered into the medical director's office and waited for him to return from lunch. And we waited. Fortunately, it was air conditioned, so it was not a bad place to wait by Liberian standards.

The medical director finally appeared, and we exchanged introductions before getting down to business. Captain Daniel politely asked about the PPE uniforms which were shipped to the Fish Town medical clinic for use in the training exercises next week. The medical director, of course, knew nothing about it. He would contact the clinic pharmacy director immediately since he was in charge of medical supply storage.

A long series of phone calls began. And we waited. And we waited some more. Meanwhile, I explained to Captain Daniel and Mark about Liberian time schedules. It is where the space-time continuum is blown apart, and there is an infinite amount of time for every little work related event in Liberian life.

Simple transactions, such as soda and bread purchases, may take 20 minutes or longer. The clerk will slowly gather the requested items and place them on the counter. You will hand him your American dollars, and he will carefully examine them as if he has never seen American currency before even though US currency is quite common here. He will then shuffle around to look for the money bucket or box (no cash registers) to give you your change. After locating said bucket/box and digging through the Liberian currency, he will discover there isn't enough change available. He will then disappear to a neighboring store to get change. Ten minutes later he will return with the correct change and slowly count out the money you are due. Meanwhile, your soda has grown warm, the bread is starting to mold, and you wish you had ordered a beer instead. Childbirth takes less time. Anyway, I digress, back to the Army.

After 45 minutes the pharmacy director arrived. We followed him back to another building and arrived at the medical supply room. He opened the door, and we entered a room packed with medical supplies such as IV fluids, medications, and PPE uniforms. Unfortunately, none of these were for the Army. The captain and I tentatively searched the corners and crevices but no luck.

Wisely, the Army brought a small supply of PPE uniforms with them so they can just reuse them during the training exercises. Since there will be no actual contact with Ebola patients during their simulated training, this will be ok. Normally, all PPE uniforms are destroyed after any exposure in an active Ebola unit.

In total, the whole process of looking for the supposedly shipped PPE uniforms consumed 1 hour and 15 minutes. The Land Rover that brought us here had departed, and we were left stranded at the medical clinic. Fortunately, we were able to contact the driver, and he returned after a 10-minute delay. We continued our tour.

We checked out the Samaritan Purse mini-ETU and the local high school where the training was to be held. We dropped the Army personnel off at the guest house where they were staying. There were 6 rooms in the guest house and 19 Army personnel staying there. The math on that was very scary. The Worst 8 Motel is looking better by the day.

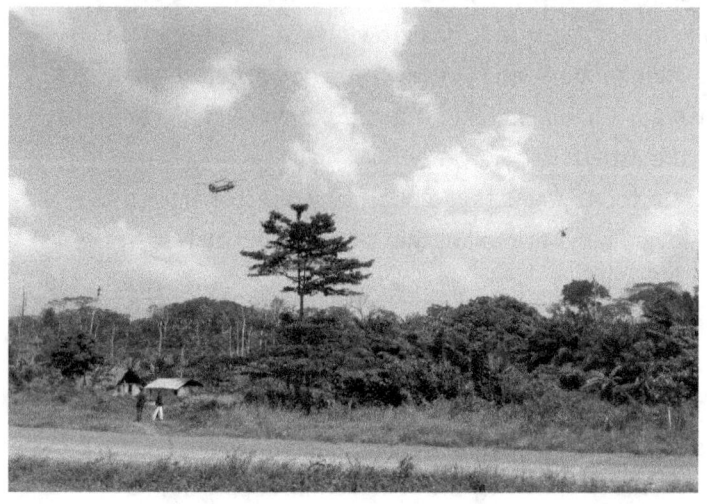

Incoming Chinook helicopters. Note house with tin roof

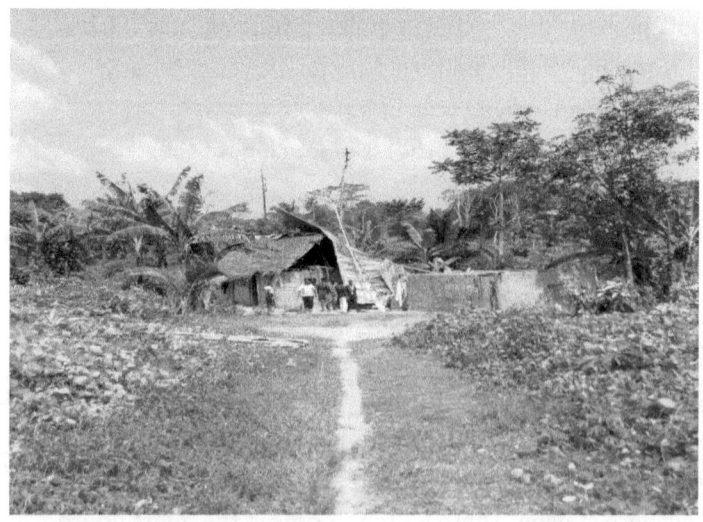

Aftermath of Chinook helicopters

The Fish Tank Opens

Our tents are up! After several delays in delivery and construction, the tents that will be our home for the next several months are move-in ready. For several days now I have been scouting the different slabs that have been poured for our tents. Our tent sites are built on the side of a hill. There are a total of ten slabs arranged in parallel pairs descending down the hill. Now I have to make the most critical decision of my Liberian trip to date...which tent to live in?

As all veteran campers know, a tent location can make or break your backwoods adventure. A swampy location or heavily wooded site with little breeze can be a feeding festival for the resident mosquitoes. A totally exposed tent site can result in near heat stroke in Texas. What you want is a spot with a scenic view, an open area for cooking, a flat area for sleeping, and some afternoon shade. A good sunset or sunrise view is also desirable.

First, I checked out the slabs at the top of the hill. These would usually be my natural choice, but they were closer to the noisy generators, furthest from the men's bathrooms, and the other tents would block the view of the jungle. Furthermore, it would catch the afternoon western sun and would be blazing hot. I ruled the top sites out.

I moved down to the very lowest sites. There were 25 yards of bare earth between the lowest slab and the perimeter bamboo fence. There was an excellent, unobstructed view of the nearby jungle. Furthermore, it faced east towards the hills and had a nice afternoon breeze. An added plus was an outside patio that caught a fair amount of afternoon shade from a nearby building. Also, the men's restrooms were on the same level, just the next tent away. My mind was made up. I staked my claim. I etched "Male Medical" in the concrete slab with an iron stake. It was a done deal.

But I was still not satisfied. I wanted not only the best tent site, but also the best bed location in that tent. A general move-in date for the masses was set for Monday. On Saturday Mark, one of our nurses, moved into a completed building in the camp, waiting for the tents to be ready. I quizzed him the next morning. He reported flushing toilets, running water, cold showers, and reliable electricity at night. I made my invasion plan.

As many friends know, I was born in Oklahoma and lived there through high school. The Oklahoma nickname is "The Sooner State." This refers to a historical event in the early 1900's when the Indian lands were first opened up for settlers. The plan was to have a land rush where a gun would go off at 7 am on the chosen date and settlers could then ride, run, walk, or drive wagons to a plot of land and stake their claim.

However, there were many not so scrupulous individuals who snuck over the night before and prematurely staked their land claim before the law-abiding citizens ever had a chance. Hence their nickname, the Sooners. This proud tradition of cheating is still carried on today by the University of Oklahoma football team.

Early Sunday afternoon I told our driver that I wanted to move into the tent camp that day. When Kelsy heard of my plans, she was also ready to go. I returned to the Worst 8 Motel for the last time to pack my bags. The driver appeared that afternoon, and Kelsy and I loaded our bags into the back of the Land Rover and started to pull out of the driveway.

One of the motel workers walked up to the back of our vehicle and knocked on the door. I recognized him as the employee who had been trying to get me to pay for borrowing the hotel's large ice cooler for the past week. I told him repeatedly that it was not my responsibility to pay and he should speak to our team manager who has continued to use the cooler. The employee continued to blame me however because I borrowed it first. I even offered to pay a rental fee of a few bucks initially, but he turned it down. I told the driver to speed up, and we left the employee in the dust. It's a cruel world.

When I arrived at the Fish Tank, my tent was up but not yet furnished with the requisite cot, mattress, and chair. It was also still dirty with dust and concrete mix on the floor. Fortunately, I had become good friends with Karmoh, the warehouse manager, and he put the hired housemaids to work cleaning and furnishing my tent while I went to dinner.

When I returned from dinner the tent was completely clean, furnished, and lighted. There were a total of seven beds available in each tent. I examined each bed carefully for view, breeze, quiet, and potential privacy. I decided on the furthest bed from the entrance. It faced the jungle and eastern horizon. It also had the most screen windows and was furthest from the social and dining rooms.

The next morning I was greeted by a beautiful sunrise streaming through my window. There was shade in the afternoon and a pleasant breeze most of the day.

I chose my roommates carefully. I invited John, a Liberian-American nurse, to take the bed next to mine. He is about the same age as me, married with four daughters, and is soft-spoken with a steady disposition. He is also Baptist and does not drink or curse, so he would be a good counterbalance to me.

I also invited Ben and Solomon, two Liberian physician assistants, who seem well educated with pleasant personalities. Both of them wish to move to America for better pay and lifestyle. They are always asking questions about American citizenship and U.S. certification for foreign trained PAs. I answer as best as I can but don't really know the specifics. I let them use my computer at night to study medical topics.

The last person who moved into our tent was Karmoh, the Liberian warehouse manager. He is usually quiet and listens to what others say. If you ask him a question about our camp, however, he will almost always know the answer. He helps me obtain supplies for my various projects around the camp, such as hammers, nails, markers, staplers, and pens. He is over 6 feet tall, very muscular, and likes to drink beer and go out to city bars at night. He is good company and protection.

So far the only downside to my tent and bed selection has been the previously unknown Muslim mosque located a few houses away. I don't know if this occurs in all Muslim mosques, but they have a very loud prayer call that goes out five times a day. I have no problem with daytime announcements, but they have a prayer call that screams out around 5 am every morning.

I am totally in support of freedom of religion, but with apologies to my Muslim friends, there should be some limitations. Why can't they just pray quietly in the early morning and forget the broadcast announcement out to the neighborhood? Every once in a while I will yell back at them that there are a bunch of Lutherans over here, and the early morning announcements are making us irritable. Apparently, they must know about Lutherans because they do not seem very worried by my threats.

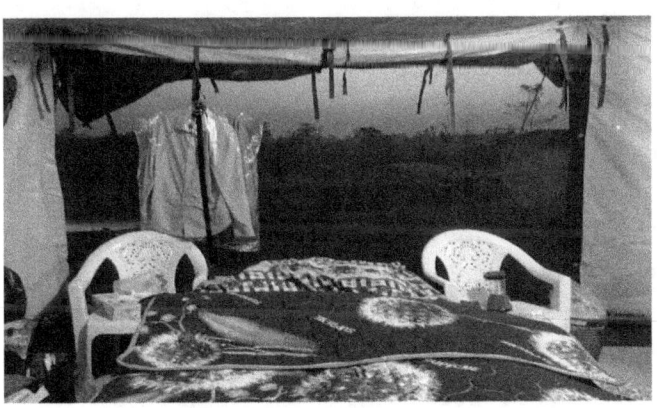

My bedroom in the Fish Tank

Furniture Fever

I have been in my tent for over a week now, and while totally satisfied with my choice, something is still missing from my life. I have been living out of suitcases for six weeks and am tired of digging through them to find certain items. I want furniture. All I have been given is a cot and a plastic lawn chair.

I scanned the grounds around my tent. There was still ongoing construction while the workers finished different building projects. I suddenly had a 70's flashback. When I was in college, living in cheap housing with little money to spare, I made furniture out of anything possible. Concrete building blocks and left over wood made fine shelves for clothing and books. I would save my money for more important items, such as beer and pot.

I looked around the grounds and saw furniture everywhere. There were left over building blocks and piles of discarded wood scattered about. I started moving concrete blocks and lumber into my tent, and soon I had fine looking 8- foot long, double shelves. I bought a laundry basket at the market, and suddenly I had a drawer for my socks and underwear.

My teammates belittled my efforts initially but were soon lusting after their own after viewing my shelving masterpiece. I had enough material left over to build shelves for my tent mates and both the cooks. I built some long shelves for Jonathan and Mark to share. I even built some shelves for Kelsy in the women's medical tent.

There is a Liberian named Benedictus who had been watching me. One day he asked to borrow my tape measure. A couple of hours later I discovered him tearing apart the large wooden shipping boxes that once contained our tents and supplies. He found a saw and a hammer and within an hour had produced a sturdy bedside table. Other team members soon joined him, and there was an assembly line producing tables and shelves. It was a defining moment of teamwork here in Fish Town. None of our appointed leaders were involved. We are strong. We are united. We are the Fish Town Ebola workers!

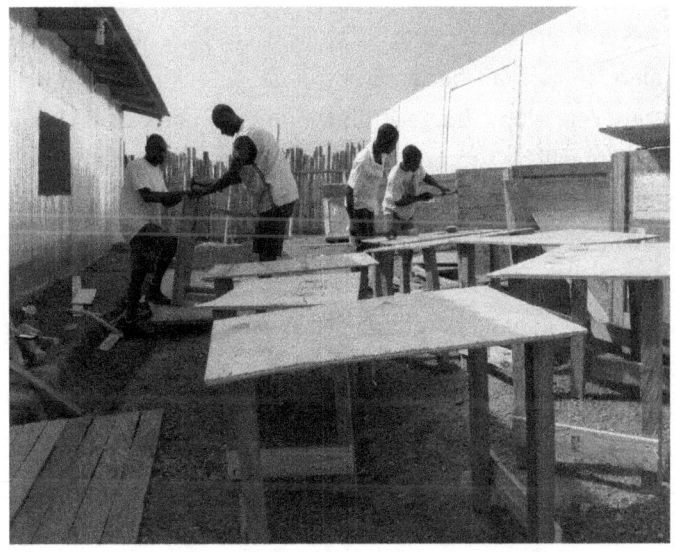

Benedictus and workers building furniture

New Year's Eve and Day

Fish Town, Liberia

New Year's Eve in Liberia is celebrated more like a religious holiday than a party. Churches have evening ceremonies, and groups of women sing traditional religious songs. Several of our Liberian nurses gathered in our social building and sang beautiful songs for a couple of hours that night. I went in to watch and hear them and was surprised to discover that even though they sang in complete harmony, they walked around separately while doing so. I have asked them to perform for us next Tuesday night at our talent show aka Liberian Idol.

New Year's Day, however, is the time to party Liberian style. There will be soccer games on satellite television all day long, and men will gather around bars and restaurants watching the games and drinking beer. When night falls things really get wild. I was invited to go downtown to Cece's, the local hang bar, by the cooks and a couple of other Liberians. Naturally, since this might involve late night hours, too much drinking, and an element of danger, I immediately accepted.

Our driver wove through the throngs of people that had spilled out of the bars and restaurants into the streets. We were finally able to squeeze into the parking lot of Cece's and join a table of jovial Liberians and a few foreigners. Afro-Pop music was blasting from a speaker as I pushed my way through the crowd to the bar and ordered the first round of drinks. I had to shout my order to the bartender who apparently could read lips because I couldn't hear myself. Women and men were dancing at their tables, in the aisles, and in the gravel parking lot. I carefully made my way back to our table while juggling drinks and dodging enthusiastic dancers.

Both of our young cooks, Reginal and Jebbeh, were dressed up with short fluffy skirts, colorful blouses, and lots of makeup and jewelry. They would spontaneously leap up from our table and begin frenzied dancing when a particularly good song blasted out. Many men would approach and try to dance with them but were usually rebuffed. A style of dancing I have seen frequently in Liberia involves the male partner humping the posterior of the female in a near rutting mode. To my older eyes it was initially vulgar, but after a couple of beers and six weeks of celibacy, it has become hypnotic and sensual. I have definitely been here too long.

I wandered out into the crowds surrounding the bar to see what else was happening. A young girl I recognized from the market approached me. I greeted her and asked her name, "Lydia." She asked if I would buy her a drink. I asked what kind of drink would she like, "Scotch." I examined her closely and asked her age, "16." Even I have boundaries, and she received a quick no.

A couple of men stopped me and asked if I would give them a job at our ETU or employee camp. I politely answered that I was not involved in the hiring process, but they persisted in giving me their names and phone numbers. Reginal found me and steered me back to our table. She told me it was not safe for me to be out in the crowds tonight. I will trust her decision.

After midnight and too many beers, the driver took me and a few others back to our camp. The party was still raging on in the streets as we made our way home. I navigated my way in the dark, on the narrow gravel pathways, and around the drainage ditches that permeate our camp to my tent and bed. I silently removed my clothes in the dark so as to not wake my tent mates and climbed into bed. I had the most restful night sleeping since moving here from Monrovia four weeks ago. I will pay for this in the morning, but it was totally worth it.

Happy New Year everyone!

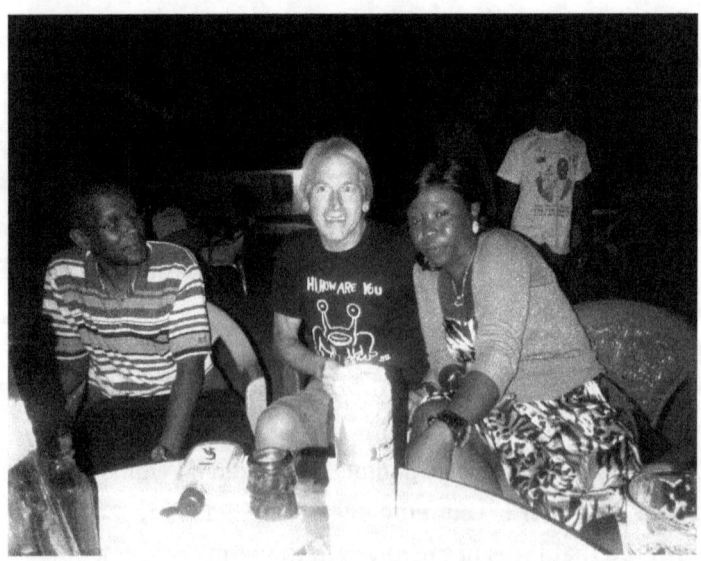

Dr. Joe and friends New Year's Day

River Gee Officials Tour Fish Tank and The Kola Nut Ceremony

We have invited the local elected and appointed officials to our camp for a tour. It was scheduled for 10 am, but of course, most officials did not arrive until almost 11 am. The mayor, who was specifically invited by our medical director several days ago, is not present. Our medical director calls her office, talks to the mayor who disavows all knowledge of the meeting but agrees to come now.

Finally, about 11 am, the meeting began. Our director thanked the officials for coming and asked if they had any questions for us. One of the officials stated he was concerned that our organization had not hired more Fish Town residents to work in our facilities. Our director rightfully pointed out that we have hired hundreds of Fish Town residents to help build our two facilities. When the facilities are completed, approximately 30 Fish Town residents will be hired to help with the ongoing cleaning, laundry, security, and cooking duties. Some will also work in our Ebola Treatment Unit as sprayers and safety directors who insure proper doffing protocol.

The official was disturbed. He had submitted a list of recommended candidates that he felt should have been used to fill these positions. Most likely this list consisted of relatives and friends of his. Our organization received over

500 applications for the 30 permanent jobs. Of these 500 applicants, promising candidates were screened, interviewed, and hired if they met the required qualifications.

The official persisted. We should have followed the local custom of hiring the individuals submitted by him. Our director replied that since lives were at stake, we would only hire the best qualified, regardless of whom they knew. This silenced him. Cronyism is alive and well in Fish Town.

They eventually got around to touring our facility. They chose my tent to visit to see what our living quarters looked like. Wisely, I temporarily took down my poster of Beyoncé, Rihanna, Ciara, and Nicki Minaj in swimsuits. I worried that the female mayor would misinterpret my intentions. I am just trying to blend into the Liberian culture. (You understand don't you June?)

I pointed to the fine desk I purchased from the local carpenter and also my makeshift curtains composed of African fabrics that I had purchased at the weekly market. I could see that she approved of my spending money in the local community. Add in my beer purchases at Cece's and Fish Town should be experiencing an economic boom.

We were later invited to a welcoming ceremony at the local government run medical clinic. We were ushered into a large conference room and awaited the medical director and others. After the required 15 minutes of waiting, the director and other officials appeared.

The director welcomed us to Fish Town. Our medical leader replied we were thankful to be here in Fish Town and offered our medical services if needed. We were to receive the historic Kola Nut Ceremony.

The kola nut is endemic to this portion of Africa and is the key ingredient used in the development of Western cola drinks. African laborers have chewed kola nuts over the centuries to diminish hunger and fatigue. When a kola nut is given to a guest, it welcomes them to a village or house. Sometimes it is a minor gesture. Other times it is a big production. Ours would be a ceremony worthy of a Hollywood production.

An emcee appeared holding a fancy ceramic plate with a single kola nut on it (a kola nut is about the size of a walnut). He held the nut up and showed it to the crowd, explaining its significance. The host placed the nut on the plate and showed it to the leader of our delegation. The leader then asked the most senior member of our delegation (unfortunately, me) to come observe and touch the plate. I then picked the nut up and passed it to our leader who held it briefly and then returned it to the plate. The plate with the kola nut on it was then paraded around the room showing it to our entire medical team. All the while the host was saying, "When the kola nut reaches home, it will tell where it came from." The proverb says that the visitor needs to show the kola nut to his people at home as proof of having visited this village. Afterwards, our medical leader and I received soft drinks as a welcome gift. Couldn't I just have had a beer instead?

Other officials from the medical center also delivered welcome speeches. Frequently, the emcee would shout out "Gbati O Gbati" with a callback by the crowd. I initially misheard this as "potty or party" and enthusiastically joined in the shout back. Later on, I was told it means "be quiet." I liked it better my way.

An elderly man appeared in a floor length gown wearing a stove top hat. We were all instructed to stand. He was the elder spokesman for the dominant tribe here, Grebo. He spoke in a strange dialect, and an interpreter translated to English. He gestured with his arms as he spoke. He welcomed us to Fish Town and River Gee County and blessed our mission. He continued for about ten minutes with frequent interruptions for applause and shout outs. He bowed to us, and we were allowed to return to our chairs. Two hours later the ceremony was finally over. I walked home, stopping at Cece's to pick up a couple of beers. It had been a long day of meetings, and I was ready for a cold shower followed by a cold beer.

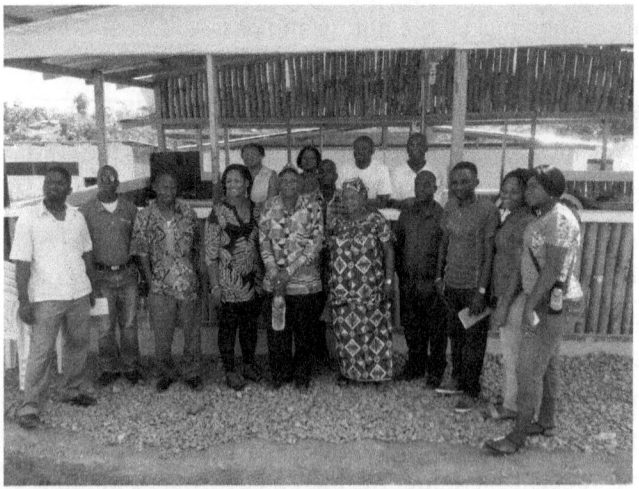

The Fish Town mayor (center, in long dress) and River Gee County officials visit the Fish Tank

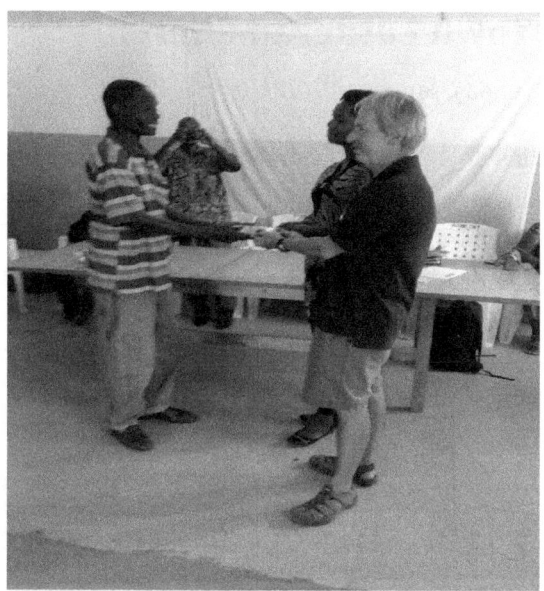

The Kola Nut Ceremony

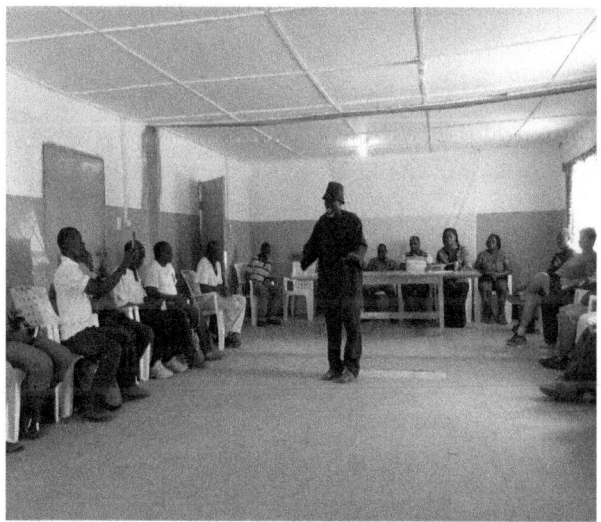

Grebo elder welcomes us to Fish Town

Fish Town Lutheran Church

Sunday, January 4th, 2015

I was walking down the main street of Fish Town last week, and a man on the back of a motorcycle hailed me and pulled over. I recognized him as Andrew, the Lutheran minister I had met briefly on Christmas Day. He thanked me for coming by the church that day and invited me to the upcoming Sunday service. He said he would like to introduce me to his congregation. I viewed this as a great way to meet the community and immediately accepted.

Kelsy, who is Lutheran, and I arrived promptly at 11 am. The service appeared to already be in progress. We sat near the front since those were the only seats available. We sat on homemade wooden benches that hold about three people across. There were some old worn hymnals beside each bench.

The minister read the story of Adam and Eve and the Garden of Eden in Genesis. He used the Socratic method of teaching, asking various members of the congregation to give their interpretation of the reading. Naturally, the snake took the brunt of the criticism. Once again, the poor creature with no arms or legs was vilified.

A collection basket was passed around, and since I had only $20 bills, I dropped one in. About 11:20 am the service was dismissed. But it was not the official service. It was the Bible study group before the service. There was much more to come.

At 11:30 a.m. the official service began. The church was now filled to capacity, and they brought in extra benches.

A young woman sat beside me and smiled.

The choir took their place along the side in lawn chairs. The choir was composed of women all dressed in colorful traditional garb with matching headpieces. There was even a percussion section with drums and tambourines. The service order was hand lettered on a poster board taped to the minister's pulpit. It followed a similar order as my Lutheran church back in Texas. I recognized the traditional confession of sin. I had come to the right place.

The service started along traditional Lutheran lines, but suddenly the choir stood and sang mightily. The ladies danced around individually and as a group while they sang in perfect harmony. There was an occasional shout out from the choir, and the congregation answered. The percussion section thumped in, and the dancers passed out castanets for audience members to join in. It was absolutely wild and very un-Lutheran-like to my way of thinking. But it was great!

At one point in the service, there was an invitation to all visitors to stand and introduce themselves to the congregation. Five of us stood, three Liberians and the two white people. Kelsy and I introduced ourselves and told them we would be working in the soon to be open Ebola Treatment Unit. The congregation clapped enthusiastically when they heard the latter.

Later on in the service, the minister announced the 2015 church budget. Wouldn't you know it, but it was our good fortune to visit on Commitment Sunday. As any good Lutheran knows, Commitment Sunday is when a member pledges to give a certain amount of money during the next fiscal year. It is something we should prayerfully consider, and a member who fails to pledge at least something to the church will leave church that day feeling guiltier than when he arrived.

Two large woven baskets were placed at the front of the church with a woman holding one basket and a man the other. The minister had wisely decided to make a contest out of it. It was the men versus the women. It was a competition I could not resist.

The choir began singing, the drums started in, and a procession of donors formed in front of the baskets. As each donor dropped his money or pledge in, the choir's singing intensified. I stood and took my place in line. I dropped in my last $ 20 and took my seat. The choir women now began frenzied dancing. I have had similar experiences back in Texas where the more money you gave, the more dancing you received, but it was definitely not in a church.

The sermon began, and it lasted an eternity. I perked up when I recognized the minister was speaking about our medical group in Fish Town. As I mentioned before, our employee camp and ETU were able to hire 30 Fish Town residents for full time positions. Unfortunately, over 500 residents applied for those 30 positions, leaving a large number of disgruntled applicants. There was a local talk radio show last week that received many unhappy calls from residents who said that our organization was not hiring local residents for jobs. The minister told the congregation that they should not be angry about not being hired. Instead, they should look at themselves to see how they could improve their qualifications for employment. It was a magical moment in our acceptance into the Fish Town community.

Kelsy and I departed early, about 1 p.m., so we wouldn't miss the camp lunch. The minister saw us leave and stepped outside the church to hail us. He thanked us for visiting today and hoped we would return. We thanked him for his kind words regarding our organization and promised to return. But next week I will arrive 30 minutes late, Liberian style.

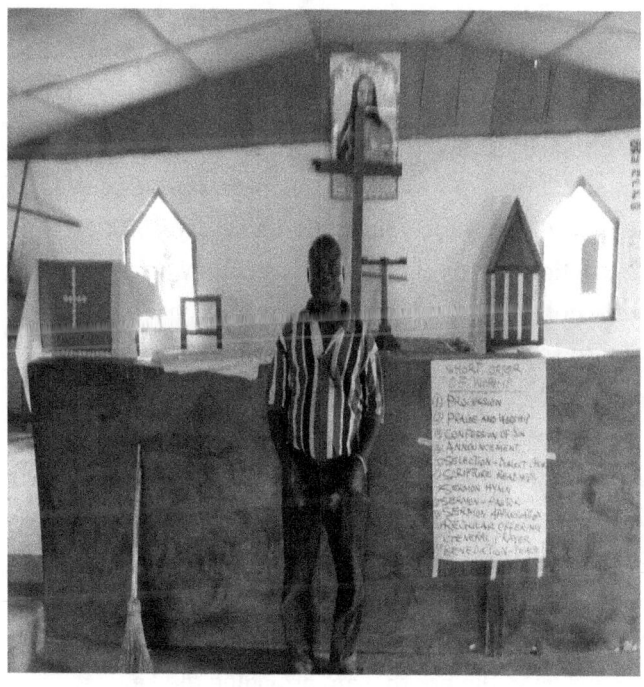

Pastor Andrew in the Fish Town Lutheran Church

Wash Your Hands!

Kelsy has come up with a brilliant idea. We should have a health fair booth at the weekly Fish Town Market. Market Day attracts thousands of shoppers and vendors, many of whom come from outlying villages. It would make an excellent venue to introduce ourselves and do a little teaching also. We decided to focus on the correct way to wash your hands. To most readers this will sound pretty silly, but in Ebola country proper hand washing can be the difference between life and death.

The Ebola virus can number in the billions per cc of blood, mucus, urine, or sweat. Person to person spread can occur explosively in densely populated areas. A 0.05% chlorine solution will kill the Ebola virus quickly and effectively, but you have to cover all the areas of your hands. To do so requires spreading your fingers and rubbing the top and the bottom of your hands. Hence, proper hand washing is an art form and is of paramount importance in the prevention of Ebola.

We reserved a booth on the front row next to the highway for maximal exposure. The nurses made a sign promoting hand washing, and we loaded up two large buckets filled with chlorinated water. A group of healthcare providers will man the booth. I am providing the key ingredient guaranteeing our success...free candy!

As soon as we arrived, I began passing out candy in a

chumming type method. Isaac, a Liberian-American nurse, took our large cardboard sign and started dancing through the crowds. A large crowd soon gathered around our booth. A line formed to learn the proper hand washing technique and, as a reward, receive some candy afterwards. We had the busiest booth in the whole market.

I took a lot of pictures for the PR folks back in Minneapolis. I strolled through the market place checking out the different items for sale. I purchased a laundry basket to use as a drawer for my homemade shelves and a new bath towel. Even though I have already purchased several yards of beautiful fabric hand made in Africa, I had to check out the latest prints.

I took several photos of children who were just too cute. The iPad was great for taking pictures and immediately showing the photo to the children. Several kids asked me to take a picture of them so they could look at the results afterwards.

We continued the hand-washing booth for over 3 hours until our relief team arrived. I walked the one-mile back to our camp, dodging killer motorcycles along the way. I heard later that our hand -washing booth was busy all afternoon even after the candy ran out. We are now planning to make it a weekly event with a different theme each time.

This was certainly not a grand humanitarian event by any stretch of the imagination, but it was a lot of fun and educational for all involved.

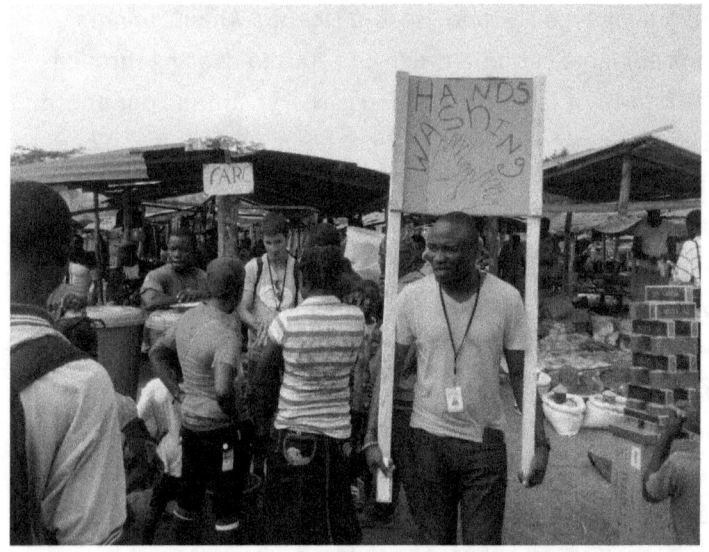

Isaac bringing in the children for hand washing school

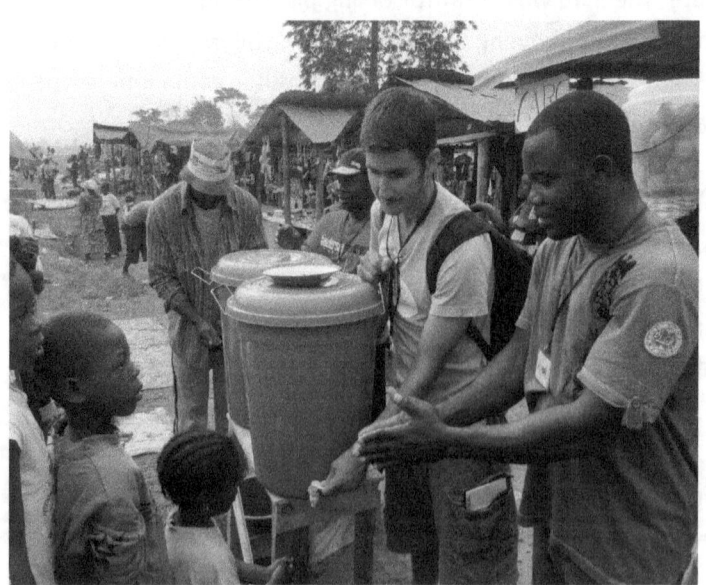

Mark teaching proper hand washing methods

White Like Me

Fish Town has a population of 3,500 people, five of which are white guys. I usually walk alone since that seems to be a better way to meet people. I pass the local carpenter, welder, bar, and City Hall every day as I make my rounds. We exchange greetings with each other and occasionally chitchat about the weather, soccer, and other local events.

As I have mentioned in past stories, I am a major draw for the younger children of which there are hundreds. They wave wildly from their yards as I pass by, frequently yelling out, "Hello White Man!" Some of the braver ones will even come out to the road and walk alongside me asking questions about my name, home, and why I am in Fish Town.

Over the few weeks I have been here, I have talked to some children repeatedly and now know their names. Many are so cute and bright that I want to take them home with me. Obviously, I have forgotten all the hard work and aggravation that goes along with raising young children. But I also miss all the joy and laughter that accompanies them. Perhaps I could just borrow them for a while?

One market day the driver had other errands to run, so he was just going to drop me off and come back to pick me up later. The weekly market attracts thousands of people and is spread out over several acres. The driver asked where he should look for me when he returned. I framed my face

with my hands and replied, "Look for the white guy."
He laughed and, sure enough, immediately found me when
he returned.

Our employee camp has been nicknamed the Fish Tank
since a chain link fence decorated with bamboo trunks
surrounds us. There are security guards in place at the two
different entrances to prevent any unlawful entries or theft.
I pass through the entry gate at least 3 or 4 times a day
when I run errands, go on walks, or go to work at the Fish
Town medical clinic. The security guards are local Fish Town
residents and have been carefully trained to look out for
possible troublemakers or thieves.

One afternoon, as I attempted to leave the camp, a
security guard stopped me. He demanded to look through
my backpack, which was suspiciously full, to be sure no
important items were being stolen from the camp. I
removed my backpack and unzipped the main compartment
to reveal...several empty large Club beer bottles! There is a
deposit on the beer bottles, and I always return the empties
when I buy full replacements. The security guard examined
the empty bottles then allowed me to exit.

I discussed this with my teammates. We decided that
in any culture there is a tendency to view minority races and
ethnic groups as outsiders and therefore, more suspicious.
Since I am white I appear most "out of place" in Liberia.
I think it is fair to generalize that if you are part of a
minority in any country or city, you can count on extra
scrutiny. Is this racism, bias, or just human nature at work?

Travel Tips for Liberia

No doubt many of my readers are now contemplating travel to Liberia in the near future. Here are a few travel tips that might come in handy as your make your way around this beautiful country.

1) Always carry water. It is always hot and humid, and you will go all day without urinating if you do not hydrate constantly. One of our physician assistants has already suffered near heat exhaustion from walking on the roads in midday.

2) Always carry toilet paper. Liberian public toilets are nasty, few, and far between, and you will be better off to just go into the jungle. Watch out for cobras while doing so.

3) Never eat food from the street vendors. See # 2

4) Wear light colored clothes that breathe. Any cotton items, such as T-shirts or jeans, will be sweated through in less than 30 minutes.

5) Always carry small bills in Liberian or US dollars. The current exchange rate is 80 Liberian dollars = 1 US dollar. If you pull out a US $20 bill or higher, you will spend half your shopping time waiting on change.

6) Always make the seller calculate the bill in both Liberian and US dollars. Most Liberians are unerringly honest, but a few will try to swindle you.

7) Never give money to beggars or you will be surrounded by a plague of others.

8) Wear comfortable walking shoes that can tolerate uneven terrain, heat, dust, chlorine baths, and torrential rains. If you find some, please let me know so I can buy a pair.

9) Always calculate delays into all appointments and travel times. Roads are impassable at times, and Liberians are never in a hurry. Relax, you are on Liberian time.

10) Always wave back at the dozens of cute, small children that wave at you as you walk and ride around town. You are a rock star. If they get close, make sure you have your wallet and valuables in your front pocket. One child will distract you in front while their accomplice sneaks up behind you to lift things out of your backpack or pockets.

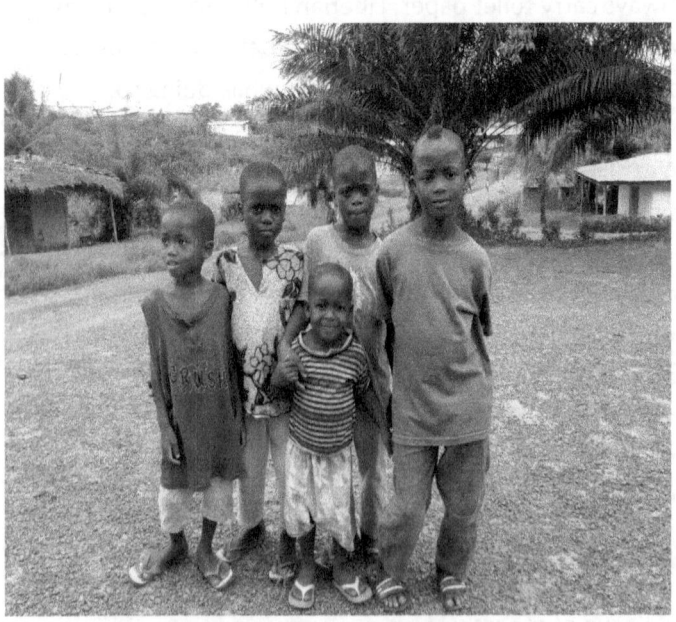

Young boys in Fish Town

Fish Tank Lecture Night

We have started a Fish Tank lecture series every Monday night. We have a diverse, well-educated group of people, and we have much to learn from each other. I have volunteered for the first lecture. It will be based on a talk I have heard several times at a medical conference, "The Ten Key Principles of All Great Leaders", by Dr. Sanjiv Chopra, a Professor of Medicine at Harvard Medical School. It is one of the most inspirational talks I have ever heard.

In the talk, ten characteristics of great leaders are covered. There is a simple mnemonic that is given:

L istening

E mpathy

A ttitude

D reaming Big

E ffectiveness

R esilience

S ense of Purpose

H umility and Humor

I ntegrity

P ack other's parachutes

I had a pretty good turnout for my lecture. There were perhaps 20 people in the room when I began my talk. I was flattered that many of them were Liberians in our group that I did not yet know well.

The Liberians were strangely silent during my

presentation. I worried that they didn't understand me with my Texas accent, but a Liberian-American later told me that native Liberians would almost always remain silent when an elder speaks. Since I am the oldest member of our party, that shut them all up.

At the end of my talk, I named several individuals who I consider to be great leaders: Gandhi, Rev. Martin Luther King, Jr., Sir Winston Churchill, Franklin Roosevelt, and Nelson Mandela. I read a passage from Martin Luther King's 1963 "I Have a Dream" speech. The Liberians were transfixed as I repeated those famous lines:

"I have a dream that my four little children will one day live in a nation where they will not be judged by the color of their skin but rather by the content of their character."

I don't think many of them had ever heard those words before. Even more mystifying, they came out of the mouth of a white man.

After my talk there was a question and answer period. One of our female doctors rightfully pointed out that I had not included any women on my list of great leaders. My bad. A Liberian nurse wanted to know if he could read the complete "I Have a Dream" speech. I showed him my iPad with the text displayed, and he studied it for 10 minutes.

Afterwards, I retired to my patio for a few beers with Jonathan, Kelsy, Mark, and a couple of my new Liberian friends. There is a radiant full moon tonight, and it is also my eldest daughter's birthday. Later on I will Skype with Ellen and nearly cry when I see her beautiful face, hear her laughter, and realize how much I miss her and home.

Happy Birthday Ellen!

How to Drive Like a Liberian

I have been in Liberia for over six weeks now and have traveled and walked the roads extensively. Having been both a passive and active participant in the travel process I feel qualified to pass on a few driving tips to anyone considering a visit to Liberia.

My first suggestion would be to forget any notion that you necessarily need to drive on the right side of the road. You should always drive on the side of the road that looks the smoothest or has the less deep pothole or mud hole. This will involve a weaving pattern of driving to achieve the smoothest ride and fastest speed possible. If there happens to be an oncoming vehicle or motorcycle you should swerve to the correct side at the last possible moment to avoid collision. If there is only one possible passage on the road, the smaller vehicle or motorcycle will yield to the larger vehicle. For those prone to motion sickness on boats and amusement rides I would definitely recommend taking a meclizine prior to travel.

If you are driving at night you should put your flashing hazard lights on. Low and high beam headlights are optional.

It is perfectly fine to pass on either the right or the left side. A warning honk is polite but not necessary.

There is a hierarchy of power and importance on Liberian roads.

1) Tankers and semi-trailers
2) Large flatbed trucks
3) SUVs
4) Small trucks and cars
5) Motorcycles
6) Goats
7) Pigs
8) Chickens
9) Pedestrians
10) Dogs

As you can see from above, people are of marginal greater significance than a stray dog if only because they make a bigger splat if you hit them.

If you should actually dare to walk on the roads you should be aware to look in both directions as you walk. Walking facing the traffic will only give you visual warning of half the vehicles trying to kill you. Be particularly alert when descending hills. Liberian motorcycle riders uniformly push their clutch in when going down hills to improve gas mileage. This will result in them silently gliding down the hill and sneaking up on you. I have had them pass inches away from me without ever hearing them.

Proper use of the car horn is essential to driving in Liberia. You should honk to pass on the left or right, if you wish to merge into traffic, if you don't like another vehicle's driving, to warn a pedestrian to get out of the way or prepare to die, or just for the sheer joy of honking.

It is rumored that in Liberian driving schools they only teach you to turn the car on, where the gas pedal is, and how to honk the horn.

Question: How do you know when a Liberian vehicle is broken?
Answer: The horn no longer works.

Things I have seen transported on a single motorcycle:
1) Five people (4 adults and 1 baby)
2) Goat
3) Pig
4) Several live chickens
5) A generator
6) A 55-gallon fuel drum (empty)
7) Mattresses
8) Sofa
9) Dining table
10) Another motorcycle

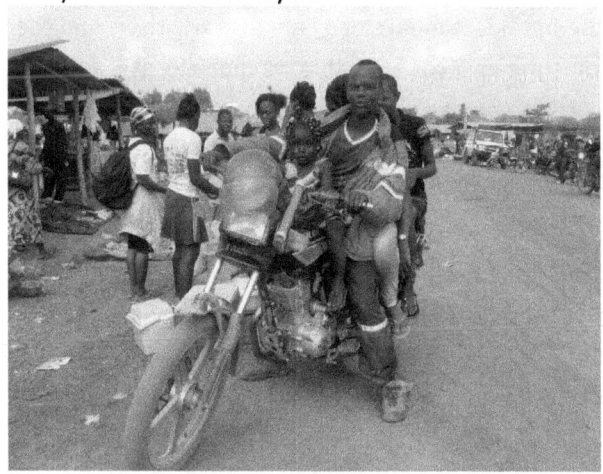

Family of 5 on a motorcycle

Cooks' Day Off

Our two cooks get up at 5 am every day to start breakfast. They prepare three hot meals seven days a week for 40 people. They work from 5 am to 8 pm preparing, cooking, and serving the food. In between they go shopping for more groceries and clean up after every meal. They were supposed to hire some relief cooks, but this has yet to happen. They are the hardest working people in the Fish Tank.

I have watched them stand outside in the hot sun and cook over the fires every afternoon. They have now worked 14 days in a row. I have decided to give them a cooks' day off.

I and several other medical personnel will cook breakfast, lunch, and dinner for an entire day. I volunteered to take the breakfast meal since I am an early riser, and the Muslim mosque ensures a reliable wakeup call at 5 am. Breakfast is also an easier meal to prepare than lunch or dinner. Despite the warm climate, Liberians like to eat hot food at every meal. I could get by with cold cereal or toast at breakfast followed by a sandwich at lunch, but that won't fly here. We must have hot rice and meat.

I have decided on pancakes, hot oatmeal, homemade bread with jam, and fresh fruit. We have a new bread maker that turns out fantastic bread. I have a whole box of pancake mix which I brought with me from Monrovia and a bottle of syrup.

I awoke at 4:30 am with the moon shining on my face. I would beat the Muslims out of bed this morning. I dressed quickly in the dark and headed for the kitchen.

The first thing I did was heat up one gallon of water for coffee and tea. As I did so, I was joined by Reuben, a Liberian nurse. I put him to work cutting up the pineapple and papaya. Doris, a Liberian-American nurse, soon followed, and she made the pancakes.

I started to make the largest batch of oatmeal ever. I filled a huge pot up with water and brought it to a boil over our propane stove. I grabbed a couple of bags of oatmeal and discovered there were no printed cooking instructions, so I just started dumping in oatmeal until the consistency seemed right. I let it boil for 10 – 15 minutes and tasted. Still a bit grainy, so I let it simmer for another 5 minutes until done.

During all of this I played Beatles and Reggae music as loud as possible on my iPad in the kitchen. We all sang along as we worked. Jimmy Cliff was a particular morning favorite.

Breakfast was on the table promptly at 7 a.m. The hotcakes sold like, well, you know. The fresh bread, butter, and jam were also a big hit. I got high fives all around. I went by the cooks' tent at 9 am to serve them the last of the breakfast, but they were still asleep. I picked up some grocery money and headed to the market.

Our first stop was the freezer trailer parked up on a nearby hill. Reuben accompanied me on the shopping trip. He has turned into a little puppy dog who follows me around since I gave my lecture on leadership last week. He has memorized the last part of Martin Luther King's "I Have a Dream" speech and quoted it to me as we walked along. His dream is to go to America, study psychiatric nursing, and become a Republican. I am glad that he has his dreams and aspirations, except, of course, for the Republican part.

We purchased 18 whole frozen chickens for $100 US. We carted the frozen chickens back home in a wheelbarrow. They will be used to make fried rice and chicken for lunch and macaroni and chicken for dinner. No cow meat today.

Next, we headed to the daily market a few blocks away. Not nearly as big in size and selection as the weekly market, nevertheless, it is the best place to shop for fresh fruit and vegetables on the other days. We were looking for fresh tomatoes and found a seller with about 30 cherry tomatoes. We purchased the entire bunch for one dollar.

All the Americans in our group lust for fresh vegetables, but all we usually find are okra and eggplant in Fish Town. None of the cabbage or cucumbers we enjoyed in Monrovia can be found. We rounded out our purchase with two large pineapples, some sweet potatoes, and whole garlic.

When we returned at 10:30 am, the cooks were awake and had resumed control of the kitchen. I turned over the produce to them and offered to help, but I was relegated to cutting up the tomatoes as a salad associate. I accepted my demotion gracefully and performed my duties without complaints.

I was completely shut out of the dinner preparations, but I saw the two cooks singing and dancing around the kitchen as they worked. That's enough reward for me.

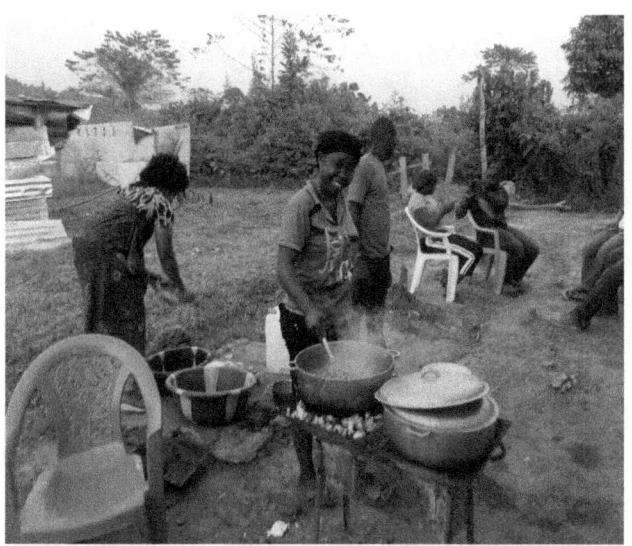

Reginal cooking up a delicious meal

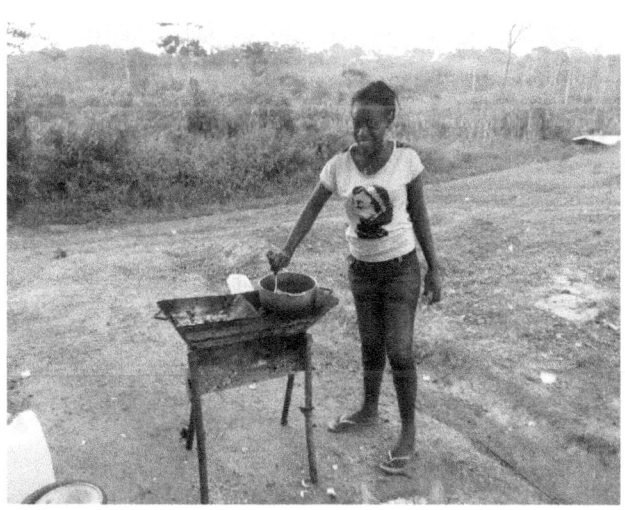

Jebbeh making a tasty dish

Fish Town Medical Clinic

Our group has been invited to the city clinic to participate in patient care on a volunteer basis. I leapt at the opportunity. I have been treating mainly upper respiratory infections, abrasions, cuts, and allergies in our medical group since we arrived in Fish Town. It has been something to do but not the real medicine I had hoped to practice in Africa.

One of our Liberian physician assistants, Soloman, a Liberian nurse, Louise, and I showed up promptly at the clinic start time of 8 am. The Fish Town outpatient medical clinic is a short 10 -minute walk from our Fish Tank camp. We introduced ourselves to the triage nurse, Denise. She welcomed us and gave us a quick tour of the clinic.

We took a look in the medical records department. It was an oversized closet filled with piles of papers stapled together. There was probably an organized system to the scattered records, but it was not visibly apparent.

There was a laboratory that performed a rapid malaria test, HIV test, typhoid test, pregnancy test, hematocrits, and blood typing. There were no chemistries, urine testing, cultures, or CBCs done here. If Ebola was a consideration, the triage nurse would send the patient directly to the temporary Ebola Treatment Unit up the road for testing and observation.   There was no radiology department here or anywhere in Fish Town. A fractured leg is put to bed and splinted. A broken arm or forearm will get you a sling for a couple of weeks. I have seen many people, both young and old, limping around town with one leg shorter than the other due to a past displaced leg fracture.

I took a look at the pharmacy. It was a dimly lit large closet with sparsely stocked shelves. The available antibiotics included amoxicillin, doxycycline, Flagyl, and trim-sulfa (Bactrim). They were out of ciprofloxacin and nonsteroidal anti-inflammatory pain medications, but those could be purchased at any number of private pharmacies around town without a prescription. There was a good selection of HIV medications and basic eye drops and ointments. There were a couple of antimalarial meds, GI antispasmodic pills, aluminum hydroxide pills for reflux esophagitis and gastritis, acetaminophen and aspirin for pain. The only antihypertensive medication they had was hydrochlorothiazide. In total, there was a bare minimum of medications available to treat common bacterial and medical problems. More complex illnesses such as tuberculosis or heart disease would require medications shipped from Monrovia or purchased from outside private pharmacies.

Prescriptions were written on a partially torn piece of white paper with the patient's name, clinic number, date of birth, today's date, along with the actual prescription orders. The same method was used for the lab orders.

There were six exam rooms: three for general medical care, one for women's health, one for mental health, and one for the eye clinic. I was given my own exam room with a bare metal exam table, lawn chairs, and an old wooden desk with many initials carved into it. One of the Fish Town clinic nurses was my assistant for the day. I recognized him from the Fish Town Lutheran Church I attended last Sunday. His name is Hamilton, and he is one of the regular nurses here.

We saw acute care patients in the morning. The patients were checked in by the triage nurse with a temperature and chief complaint. They were then directed to the appropriate clinic, be it the women's, general medical, or eye clinic. The chart was pulled and placed on the doctor or nurse's desk, and the patients lined up in the hallway in the order in which they presented.

The first patient I saw was a 7- year-old girl with headache, fever, and chills for several days. The young girl was lethargic and appeared ill. I examined her, and the only notable finding was splenomegaly, a common finding in malaria. I sent her to the lab, and the rapid blood test for malaria was positive. I prescribed a weight appropriate dose of antimalarial medication for several days and Tylenol. I saw a 10- year-old girl with similar symptoms; she too had malaria.

An elderly male came in with a several day history of nausea, vomiting, and lower abdominal pain. He had a large right inguinal hernia that was tender to touch. I was able to gently reduce it, and his discomfort subsided. I asked him to wait around a few hours before going home to be sure the hernia had not compromised the blood flow to a portion of his intestine. He was able to drink some water, kept it down, and was allowed to return home. He was scheduled for surgery the next week. A middle-aged male came in with an asymptomatic left inguinal hernia. I ordered pre-surgical lab to include malaria testing, hematocrit, and blood typing.

I saw an 18- year-old girl with fever, myalgia, and painful swallowing. These are all symptoms of Ebola, and my radar went up. I wore gloves to examine her and found tender submandibular lymph nodes. I looked inside her throat and saw bilateral enlarged, reddened tonsils covered with a white exudate. She had strep throat, not Ebola. I gave her some amoxicillin and Tylenol and sent her on her way.

Another young woman in her 20s had been having lower abdominal pain and fever the past few days. I examined her and found bilateral adnexal masses and tenderness. Rose, the Women's Health Clinic midwife, came over and confirmed my findings. We concurred that the patient probably had PID (pelvic inflammatory disease), an infection frequently caused by gonorrhea. I prescribed one large dose of Flagyl followed by several weeks of doxycycline.

I saw about twelve patients over the morning, including many young children with upper respiratory infections. A middle-aged woman came in complaining of palpitations. She had a past history of hypertension but was not taking medications for such. There was no blood pressure cuff. They had all been removed since the Ebola epidemic. I took her pulse, which was 80 and regular, and listened to her heart and lungs; they sounded fine.

Hamilton told me to give her two weeks of hydrochlorothiazide and send her home. I told him that in the United States we usually give antihypertensive medications on a daily basis. The nurse replied, "Yes, I know, but that is not how we do it here. You give the medications until the symptoms subside and then you stop." Hmmm, interesting concept. I have seen many of my noncompliant patients do the same in the United States, so maybe it works.

We finished around 12:30 p.m. I picked up my stethoscope and backpack and prepared to leave. Rose, the Women's Clinic midwife, stopped me to ask if I would like to come back next week and work with her in the Women's Clinic. Apparently, she was impressed with my PID findings. It has been a while since I've provided women's healthcare, but it is better than building furniture or hauling water to fill our water tanks, so I accepted.

Hamilton also stopped me and took me back to our exam room. He first asked for money for his Lutheran church and then money for himself. I told him I only have a limited amount of money for my stay in Fish Town but will think about his church when I return home.

Our medical group has had ongoing discussions regarding our plans and activities while awaiting the opening of our Ebola treatment unit. Our medical director keeps talking about "sustainability." She downplays my work at the Fish Town medical clinic, saying it is only temporary help that will disappear with my departure and will not have a long -term impact on Fish Town or Liberia.

I have been thinking about the concept of sustainability. What money or actions can you pour into such an impoverished country as Liberia that will make a long-term difference? I accept that the medical work I provide here is only temporary. I could say the same thing about the medical work I provide in Texas. My patients will age and die over time no matter what I do. It is a simple fact of life that all services we provide to each other are only temporary.

I believe that any act of kindness and human concern is always worth the effort. To relieve human suffering on a personal basis is of great value to the person receiving the services. If what I am doing here is just pissing in an ocean of human misery, I would just as soon go ahead and piss.

My day at the Fish Town medical clinic has been the most rewarding and satisfying day I've had since arriving in Liberia. I was allowed to see and examine patients, order lab tests, and prescribe medications. I am finally making a difference in Liberia. If I am allowed to continue seeing patients at the Fish Town medical clinic, my trip will be justified.

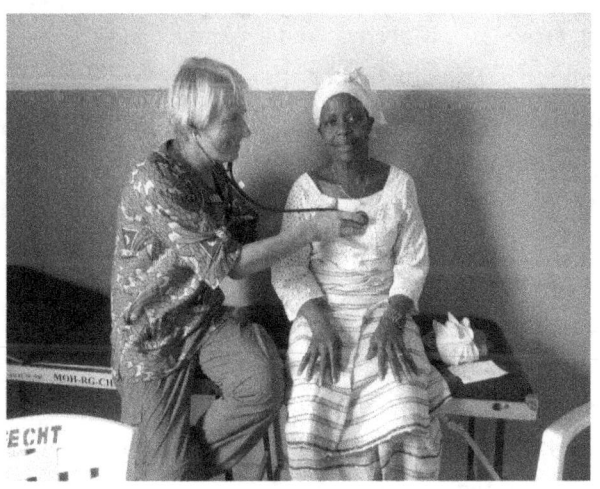

Dr. Joe at work at the Fish Town medical clinic

Fish Town Women's Clinic

I have worked in the general medical clinic for two days, and Rose, the Women's Clinic midwife, has now invited me to come work with her. I have not done any obstetrics in many years, but Rose appears young and enthusiastic about her work as opposed to the older general medical nurse who rarely touches patients and blindly treats diseases based on history alone. On the second day I worked in the general medical clinic, the nurse briefly came in, noted I was there with one of my team nurses, and left for the rest of the day. Government workers, they're all alike.

Rose is in her early 30s and has been a midwife for 4 years. During that time she has delivered over 1,000 babies. Midwife certification in Liberia requires two years of school, an apprenticeship, and successful completion of a certifying exam. Rose grew up in Monrovia and accepted the government job in Fish Town right after graduation. She dreams of being an Ob-Gyn doctor, but it will require another four years of college followed by four years of medical school.

There are hundreds of young kids in Fish Town. After spending a few days in the Women's Clinic, I know where they all come from. Young women from ages 14 to 20 are the bulk of our patients. Birth control is rarely practiced, and young girls are fair game for all males. The young mothers are rarely married and are lucky to even be living with the father of their child.

But there are plenty of older pregnant patients too.

We see women in their 20s and 30s who have had 6 to 10 pregnancies. Although there are some Catholics in town, religious beliefs don't seem to be the reason why people are having so many children. Copulation seems to be the major activity for couples at night. These people desperately need cable TV.

Rose is a patient teacher. She showed me how to measure the height of the pregnant uterus. The height of the fundus in centimeters roughly correlates with the number of weeks for the pregnancy. (I apologize to my Ob-Gyn colleagues if I am completely off base here. Hey, I'm an Internist in Africa.)

We used a primitive stethoscope to listen for fetal heartbeats which are audible at 20 weeks of pregnancy. I have even learned to locate the head of the baby to make sure it is in the right position for delivery. How cool is that?

You might ask, "Joe, couldn't you easily do all that with a simple ultrasound?" And I would reply, "Yes, but we are in Fish Town, Liberia, where the possibility of having an ultrasound is less likely than the chance of being invaded by space aliens." And therein lies the challenge and the excitement of practicing medicine in a third world country. It is back to the basics with your eyes, ears, hands, and most of all, your mind.

Rose showed me how to insert implants into a patient for pregnancy prevention. Then I performed the procedure on the next three patients. It is a relatively simple procedure. First you numb the upper inner arm with subcutaneous lidocaine, then you insert a large bore needle just under the skin for several inches, and then the implant is passed through the middle of the needle much like you would load the muzzle of a gun. It was another first in my medical career. Better late than never.

On my first day with Rose, we worked from 8 am to 3 pm without a break. There was a continuous stream of pregnant women into our office. There were frequent interruptions as the triage nurse, lab technician, and pharmacist entered for questions or results. Through it all Rose remained calm and collected.

There was a 39-year old pregnant woman who had both malaria and newly diagnosed HIV. Despite the fact that we had been working without a break for seven hours, Rose slowed down, closed the door to all interlopers, and empathetically explained HIV disease. She reassured the patient that she and her baby would be fine with the right medications and careful follow-up care. Call the medical care in Liberia substandard if you will, but in my estimation the actual care practiced by Rose was first rate.

One afternoon, a man rode up on the back of a motorcycle holding a young boy who was having a seizure. Rose was there and quickly assessed the young boy. She thought the boy had cerebral malaria and ordered the father to take the child to a nearby hospital. The father ran back out with the seizing child, jumped on the back of a waiting motorcycle, and raced off to the hospital.

Cerebral malaria is a known complication of P. falciparum, the most common type of malaria in Liberia. It can be treated with antimalarial drugs and the seizures controlled with Valium or Ativan. Most children with cerebral malaria will recover, but a few will be left with permanent neurologic deficits, such as paralysis, poor coordination, and epilepsy, and some will die.

During my 30 years of medical practice in Texas I've only seen two cases of malaria. Both patients had contracted their disease in the jungles of Mexico or Central America. Since arriving in Fish Town one month ago, I have diagnosed two dozen cases of malaria.

Malaria is most common and severe in children between 5 to 12 years of age. As Africans age they may have subsequent infections, but they are not as severe as the initial one.

A member of our staff, who has visited Africa multiple times in the past, became ill with fever and rigors last week. I treated him for malaria with Malarone, the same medication I have been taking for prevention. This is also the best medicine for treating P. falciparum but is considered too expensive for widespread use in Africa..

Today, while working the general medical clinic, a 62-year-old woman came in complaining of post-menopausal bleeding and abdominal pain. She had been seen two other times in the medical clinic and was given antibiotics for a presumed infection, but she did not improve.

I examined her abdomen and felt a mass in either her left ovary or uterus. Fortunately, that was the first and only day our medical director had brought her portable ultrasound machine to the clinic, and we were able to use it on this patient. And yes, there was a large pelvic mass present. The woman is now scheduled for a hysterectomy. Pissing in the ocean of human misery is my business.

Incident Report

January 17, 2015 Fish Town, Liberia

At 6:30 this morning I was sitting in our outdoor dining room when a security guard approached me. He said there was a woman outside our gate requesting assistance for another woman who had collapsed at a nearby house.
I grabbed my stethoscope, exam gloves, a flashlight, and followed the woman down a nearby road. As I approached the house, I could see a woman lying on her back in the dirt entranceway. A man was supporting her head.

The woman was conscious but responded weakly to questions and commands. The surrounding witnesses said the woman had complained of lower back and abdominal pain early this morning. When she tried to stand up, she said she was dizzy and then fell to the ground.

There was no history of recent trauma. I was able to elicit a history of no menstrual periods for two months, and the good possibility that she was pregnant. She denied nausea, vomiting, diarrhea, fever, or chills. She was 28 years old and was previously in good health.

When I examined the patient she was awake but followed commands poorly. Her pulse was 100 and weak. Her neck was supple, lungs clear, and heart sounds were normal. I felt her uterus approximately 3 cm above the pubic bone. There was no upper abdominal tenderness. On palpation of her back, I could not elicit tenderness. She was able to weakly move her legs.

My assessment was that of a young, pregnant female with the sudden onset of abdominal and lower back pain, followed by dizziness and weakness.

The possible etiologies included:

-ruptured ectopic pregnancy, but that would not explain the palpable uterus.

-miscarriage or spontaneous abortion.

--ruptured ovarian cyst or follicle.

- some other abdominal or pelvic process.

We laid her on a mattress, and I asked a family member to call the hospital or ambulance service. This request was met with blank faces. No one had a cell phone. No one had a motorcycle or vehicle.

I quickly returned to our nearby compound. When I passed through the gates, I saw Lawrence, one of our drivers. I told him about the sick woman who needed immediate transfer to the hospital. He recruited another male, and they climbed into a Land Rover and drove off to retrieve the woman. A few minutes later I walked out of our compound and observed the Land Rover racing by with the woman inside.

Sincerely,

Joe Spann, M.D.

Follow up Jan. 28th, 2015

The woman was safely transported to the Fish Town Hospital where she was admitted for several days. I did not get all of the details, but she received some IV fluids and blood products and was able to go home without having surgery.

There was another call for emergency transportation to the Fish Town Hospital that same morning, but there were no hospital ambulances available. To their credit, Lawrence and the other ARC employee drove out with the Land Rover and transported that patient back to the hospital. A two-for-one rescue effort by ARC employees in the Fish Town community. We are making an impact, one person at a time.

A week or so later I was walking past the woman's house, and she came out to thank me. She reported feeling well and was looking forward to having another child. I did not get a picture of her, but I did take a picture of her children in front of their mud brick house.

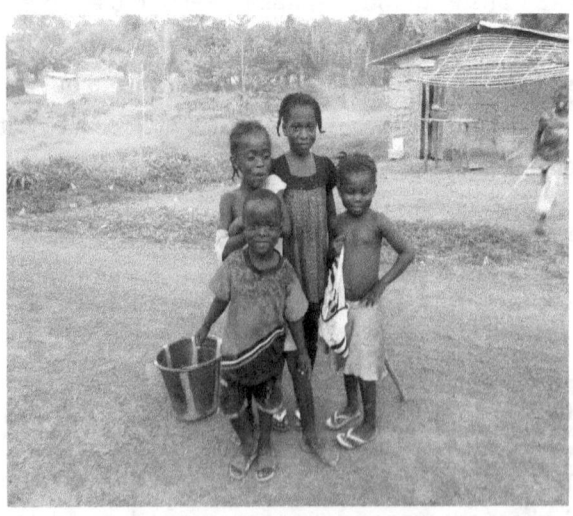

Children in front of their home

Planned Parenthood of Fish Town, Liberia

Rose has invited me to speak at the weekly meeting of the Planned Parenthood Association of Fish Town. She is the president and is interested in outside speakers. I am about the most outside speaker you can get.

Most of the previous lectures have been about teenage pregnancy, sexually transmitted diseases, violence towards women, rape, drugs, and alcohol abuse. The audience will be primarily teenagers that Rose has mentored over the past few years.

I have decided to repeat my lecture on leadership because I believe the Fish Town community is in need of good leaders. What I have seen so far from the Fish Town and River Gee elected and appointed officials is cronyism and elitism. Fish Town needs an honest leader who can bring sustainable business and jobs to a community that sorely needs such.

My lecture was scheduled for a Tuesday afternoon at 4 pm. I had a very busy day at the Fish Town medical clinic prior to the lecture. I raced home at 3:30 p.m. to take a quick shower and retrieve my hand lettered poster board. I bought a bag of candy, several bags of popcorn, and a large package of Oreo cookies to give out to the kids.

I arrived at the Planned Parenthood Association of Fish Town just before 4 pm. There was sheet metal fencing surrounding the tiny building with a swinging wooden door as the entrance. Rose had put up handwritten signs outside announcing my lecture. Liberians rarely have middle names, so she gave me the abbreviated name of "Dr. Joseph Logan." That was ok with me because I usually just go by Dr. Joe.

Rose greeted me and showed me to the lecture room, which was a room the size of a small bedroom. It was packed with older children and teenagers in lawn chairs talking with each other. I estimated about 25 kids altogether with a wide range of ages. I placed my large poster board atop a desk against the back wall for better viewing.

Rose ordered silence in no uncertain terms, and the kids immediately quit talking. She introduced me to the audience as a doctor from America who had come to fight Ebola (okay, so I'm not exactly fighting Ebola at the moment. Sounds heroic.)

I made an effort to slow down my words so that the Liberians could understand me. I thanked them for inviting me to their meeting and asked them to please raise their hand if they had trouble understanding me or had questions.

Younger Liberians are traditionally very reticent to ask questions of elders (yep, that's me) and usually sit quietly during lectures. This is somewhat unsettling as a speaker, especially if you are trying to tell a joke. I have tried delivering a humorous line a couple of times when speaking to groups in Liberia and have been universally greeted with stone silence. Ok, I admit some of my jokes aren't that funny.

I went through my lecture emphasizing honesty, hard work, empathy, and a sense of purpose. Since it was Planned Parenthood, I also emphasized the need to NOT get pregnant when you are young to the girls. If they are to be leaders, they will need to stay in school instead of becoming teenage mothers. I followed that with a direct message to the boys in the room. They too needed to avoid teenage pregnancy if they were to realize their dreams. They should be as equally responsible as the girls.

We discussed great leaders in history. They knew very little about American or British figures but have heard of Martin Luther King, Jr. and Nelson Mandela. I recited a few sentences from the "I Have A Dream" speech, and they were mesmerized by those immortal words.

There was a question and answer period after my lecture. A high school boy complained that both of his parents were dead, and he now lived with his grandmother who had little money. He wanted to go to college but could not afford it.

I know little about Liberian colleges, tuition, student loans, or scholarships. I told him that my father went to college and worked washing dishes in a rooming house to pay for his housing and tuition. Anything is possible if you believe in yourself and work hard.

One teenage boy stood up and addressed me as "White Man." Rose quickly corrected him and told him to call me Dr. Joe. I answered his question and concluded with, "Do you understand Black Man?" That got a lot of laughs from the kids. Point made.

There had been an adult standing in the doorway during most of my lecture. After I finished, Rose introduced me to Michael, a news reporter for the local (and only) radio station in town. He enjoyed my lecture and wanted to interview me for his morning radio show. I hesitated initially because I hate live interviews in the early morning. He clarified by stating the interview would be right then and recorded for the morning show. Much better.

So I did the interview and rehashed most of my major points on good leaders. He asked why I would speak to teenagers and children when I could be talking to adults. I told him that these children and teenagers would be the future leaders, so they were the most important people in town. He liked that response and promised to air my interview in the am.

I passed out the candy, popcorn, and cookies after the lecture, and many pictures were taken of Rose and the kids. Rose walked me home and thanked me for coming. I, in turn, thanked her for letting me be a small part in her attempt to change the culture of Fish Town.

My interview played on Fish Town radio the next morning about 7:30 a.m. Apparently, everyone in town listens to the local radio broadcast in the morning. All day long I was approached by strangers who enjoyed my interview and who thanked me for coming to Fish Town. It was another unexpected surprise in a trip that continues to amaze me.

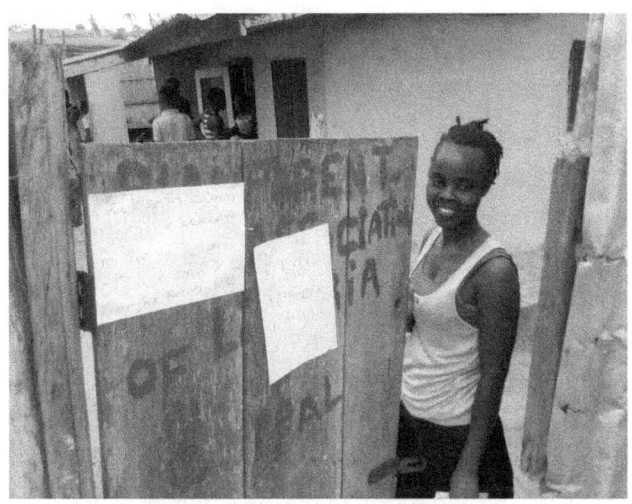

Rose at Planned Parenthood of Fish Town

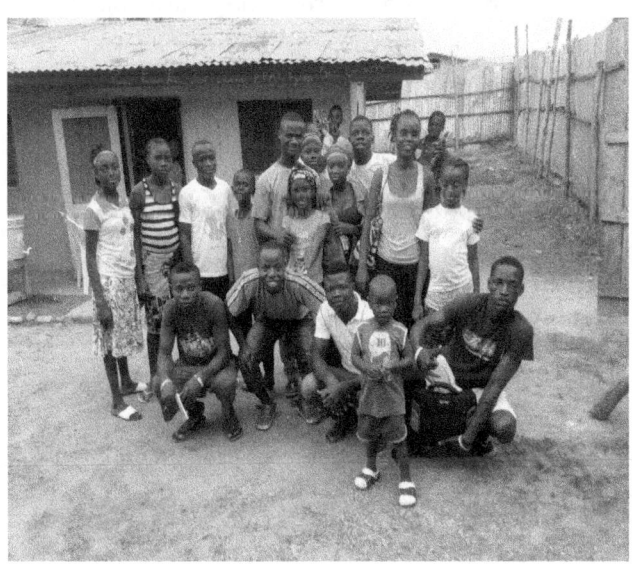

Rose and her students at Planned Parenthood

My First African Birthday

I awakened at 5:30 am as is my habit now in the Fish Tank. The Muslim mosque makes a pretty good alarm clock, and I have made my peace with them. I walked past the mosque the other night and discovered several of our Liberian workers awaiting prayer services. They are kind people. Although their prayer calls are a bit noisy, I will let it slide.

I enjoy the solitude and quiet of the early morning. The steady rumble of the generator keeps me company along with the crowing of an occasional rooster. It is also the coolest part of the day. The days are getting warmer and more humid now as we head towards the summer. The nights are also warmer than they were a couple of weeks ago. We still have the haze of the Sahara sand most days, but it is lessening. It hasn't effectively rained in weeks, and the roads are especially dusty now. When I walk along the road, I turn my head and cover my mouth and nose to block the flume of dust that follows every passing vehicle and motorcycle.

At breakfast this morning the cooks, Reginal and Jebbeh, presented me with a bottle of wine and a beautiful green and black African style shirt. They appreciated my attempt to give them a day off a couple of weeks ago. We also share the same party attitude with dancing and drinking on the weekends at Cece's bar; although, I do most of the paying, and they do most of the drinking and dancing.

Mark arrived and carved up a fresh pineapple for

breakfast, writing a large announcement on our daily activity board, "Dr. Joe's Birthday!" We had one of my favorite meals, fresh baked bread, for breakfast. I was treated to the first round of "Happy Birthday" sung by an enthusiastic crowd of early morning risers. We are a captive group here at the Fish Tank, and mine is the first birthday celebrated since we moved in.

I am off to church this morning. I have decided to visit the church Rose attends. It is just down the road from our camp, and the service starts at 10:00 am. The church is named Dominion Christian Fellowship Center and to my knowledge isn't associated with any specific denomination.

I arrived promptly at 10:00 am, so that meant I was the only person present in the church. Eventually, Rose showed up, other people arrived, and the service began. It was not the actual service but rather a Bible study. It was now too late to gracefully withdraw, so I sat down for the class.

Today's topic was the difference between a vow, an oath, a pledge, and a promise. I hadn't really thought about the difference before, and I was intrigued. I reason that a marriage vow is something that is taken in the presence of friends, family, and God. So a vow must be a promise to God and others. An oath would be like the Hippocratic Oath I took when I became a doctor. I remember, "First do no harm," so I think it must be a promise I make to society. But then you also take an oath when you testify in court, and it ends with "so help me God," so maybe there is a promise to God involved also. The Pledge of Allegiance must be a promise you make to a country or flag, and a plain promise is something you make to another person or business.

There was an hour -long discussion back and forth in our group. I'm not sure if they understood my Hippocratic Oath or Pledge of Allegiance references, but they seemed to enjoy my participation in the dialog.

A little after 11:00 am there was a short break before the real service started. I had been drinking lots of tea and water that morning and looked for a mythical public restroom. Unbelievably, there were public restrooms directly behind the church, but all the doors were padlocked. I ducked behind the restroom to do my business and immediately saw a female with the same idea. She politely backed off, and I was allowed to proceed. After washing my hands in the chlorine mixture for preventing the spread of Ebola, I went back inside the church for the big show.

And what a show it was! If I thought the Fish Town Lutheran Church was a hot performance, the Dominion Christian Church was a show in Las Vegas! There were two choir groups composed of women, an older group and a younger group. The service began with the two choir groups singing, clapping, and snaking their way into the room for over 10 minutes before finding their chairs along the side. There were short periods of time when the assistant or pastor spoke, then the choir would spontaneously erupt in song, and the dancing and shout outs began anew.

Rose is a superstar in her church. She sat up next to the pastor and the band (drums and organ). She frequently stood up to start many of the songs. She strolled down the main aisle in song, the choir jumped in, the band started thumping out a rhythm, and we were off for another 10 minute throw down show.

There was a hyperactive kid sitting directly behind me on a wooden upright bench. He nervously kicked and touched my backside during most of the service. It was not painful but bothersome nonetheless. I turned several times and smiled politely, but he must have been alone because the kicking and hitting soon started up again. I chose to ignore this mild distraction.

At certain points in the service there would be a shout, and all the members started talking nonsensically to themselves. It was the mystical "speaking in tongues" I had heard about but never witnessed. Fortunately, or unfortunately, there was no snake handling involved.

There was the introduction of visitors and about a dozen stood. There were several other members of our medical team present, but I was the only white person. The congregation applauded as each individual gave their name and home. I usually give Texas as my home and am generally greeted by silence. Rarely, somebody will know something about cowboys or Texas that they learned from watching movies or TV and will ask me questions afterwards.

The pastor gave his sermon with incredible enthusiasm that was mirrored by the congregation's response. I can't tell you what he was speaking about, but it sounded very motivating. Even after being in Liberia for two months, I still have difficulty understanding what the natives are saying. The Liberians use a type of shorthand in their words using predominantly nouns and verbs so their sentences come out very clipped and abbreviated. A typical interview question for a medical appointment would be, "What be bothering you?" I am embarrassed to admit that I usually have a Liberian staff member with me to help communicate with my Liberian patients. My American teammates like to tease me saying that it is the Liberians who are really suffering trying to understand my "Texas English".

After the one-hour sermon, there was more singing and dancing, and the offering process began. You are given a piece of folded construction paper that will be used as an envelope. Rows of the congregation are led up to a large basket at the front of the church and individuals drop the offering in. As the money accumulates, the singing and dancing becomes more frenzied. It is an idea I should export to my own Lutheran church back home in Austin.

The service finally ended a little after 1:00 p.m. I stood up to leave, and Rose appeared to lead me outside. I thanked her for inviting me, said goodbye, and began my short walk home. A young girl in a pretty dress joined me and started a conversation. Her younger brother held my hand as we walked. They lived in a house not too far from our camp and saw me walking by nearly every day. The young girl asked my name and where I was from. Her name was Cecelia, and she wanted to know more about my medical group and America. We talked for a short while as we walked towards their house. She wanted to come visit our camp someday, and I told her I would try to arrange it. I'm not sure what my superiors would say about bringing a young girl to our camp, but it seemed like a good way to take the mystery out of our walled off compound.

I dropped them off at their house and returned to my

camp for lunch. There was another round of the "Happy Birthday" song as we ate. Afterwards, I answered some e-mails, wrote a little, and took a brief, sweaty nap.

At 4 p.m. it was time for our first game of Ultimate Frisbee. Mark loves this activity and had recruited three of us to go to a nearby soccer field to play. Surprise, surprise, there were soccer teams already playing there. As we walked back on the road, I playfully tossed the Frisbee to a couple of curious children. The kids had never seen a Frisbee and were totally enthralled. Mark taught them how to throw the Frisbee, and they were soon making good tosses and catches.

More kids were drawn in by the Frisbee activity. We moved over to the large front yard of an empty building and started tossing the Frisbee back and forth with the new arrivals. Before I knew it there were at least 50 kids chasing and throwing the Frisbee. Fights started breaking out over control of the Frisbee. The parents of the children gathered on the perimeter to watch the activity. The sight of four white adults surrounded by a mob of shouting, delighted Liberian children is a surreal moment I will not soon forget.

We had to stop the Frisbee game after several small children were trampled by others when they attempted to get the Frisbee. We walked home to our camp with a mob escort. I got them to start marching in formation and singing military cadence songs. Mark even got them to sing the "Happy Birthday" song to me one more time.

We were served spaghetti with tomato sauce, chicken, and shrimp for dinner. It is my favorite meal here at the Fish Tank. One more round of the "Happy Birthday" song and it was time for libations. We gathered on my patio for beer and wine. I was given a homemade birthday card from my American teammates with many nice things written in it. I felt totally undeserving of their kind words and respect. Later on in the night, I Skyped with my wife, daughter Amy, and my sister Lisa in California.

It was a wondrous birthday, especially considering my last birthday. My mother had died 3 days prior, and the idea that I should celebrate an occasion when the person who made it all possible was no longer alive just didn't seem right. As it turned out, my mother had already purchased a birthday card for me as if she knew she would not be there to give it to me. So Mom.

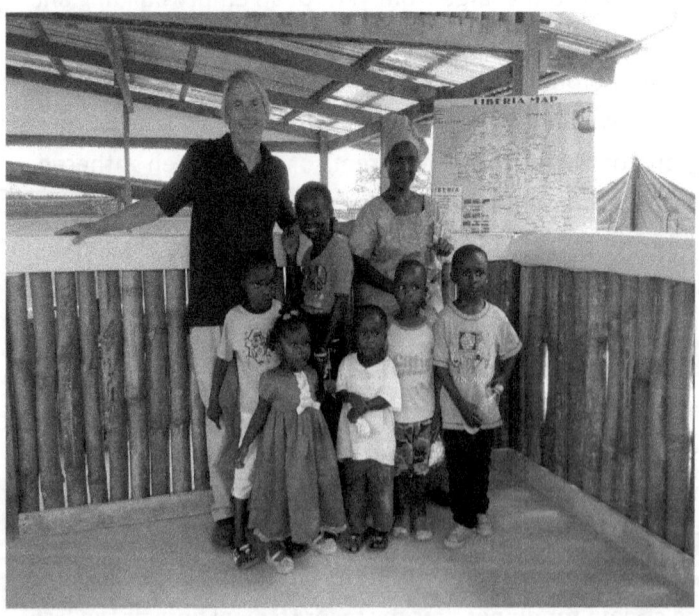

My neighbors next door

Machete Wars

Machetes are quite common in Liberia and are used for a variety of purposes. They are used to mow the grass, kill snakes, cut up pineapples and coconuts, for general carpentry, and for clearing land. Machetes are the Liberian equivalent of Swiss Army knives. They can be purchased at most stores in Fish Town for about $6 to $8, depending on size. It is not uncommon to see a young boy about 8 or 10 years old walking down the road carrying a machete that is half his size.

Kelsy has been eyeing the machetes for quite some time and has decided to buy one to take back to her Minnesota cabin. Jonathan, our Montana nurse, has heard of her plan and has also decided to purchase a machete for himself.

Upon further thought, Kelsy has decided two additional machetes will be required for her two nephews, ages 10 and 12. Over several beers on my porch, we debated the wisdom of giving machetes to the two young boys. The older boy is certainly capable of safely handling a machete, but there was some uncertainty about the younger brother. We decided it would definitely be unfair for the younger boy to not have a machete, and we approved both boys as machete worthy.

We then considered the father of these young boys and whether he should have a machete too. Certainly in the line of machete power, he should definitely have a bigger machete. The father is also approved for a machete.

Kelsy was now up to a total of four machetes for potential purchase. Jonathan had been following closely and has now developed a bad case of machete envy. He decided he must purchase machetes for all of his nephews. The nephews range in age from 5 to 16 years old, and they must all have machetes.

I attempted to perform an intervention. I told them both that when they return to the United States and are screened at the airport, the authorities would note that they were Ebola workers returning from Liberia with multiple machetes in their suitcases, and they would be locked up for 90 days instead of the usual 21 days. This did not seem to deter them.

I myself plan on purchasing only a single machete for personal use, unless of course, my daughters, wife, brother, nieces, or nephews decide they need one. Perhaps I can negotiate a big discount for a mass purchase?

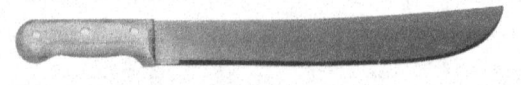

Doctor Joe

Fish Town, Liberia

The Ebola epidemic of 2014 – 2015 is essentially over. There have been no reported Ebola cases in River Gee County where I am stationed for over 60 days. There have only been 4 – 5 cases of Ebola in the entire country of Liberia the past two weeks. Our twenty bed ETU is finally nearing completion, but there are no patients for it.

We are not the only ETU facing this reality. Hundreds of healthcare workers have poured into Liberia and other neighboring countries to fight Ebola, but we have arrived just in time for the end. We are sitting in million dollar camps and ETU units with little to do but rehearse for Ebola patients that may never arrive.

I have finally convinced our medical director that going out to the local medical clinics and providing primary care is important to the patients and our staff. She still encourages "sustainability" as an all-important goal, but we need to see patients for our own sense of worth and sanity. If we can't treat Ebola patients, can we at least treat some patients?

I have become a regular fixture at the Fish Town medical clinic. I have my own exam room and a rotating group of nurses and PAs that work with me. I arrive about 8 am and start seeing patients around 9. I see about 20– 25 patients a day ranging in age from 5 to 80 years old.

I have become fairly adept at diagnosing malaria, one of the most common illnesses in Fish Town. Most of the malaria patients are young, 5 – 15 years of age, and have a history of fever and chills for 1-2 days. The exam will be notable for a fever and a palpable spleen. The confirmatory lab test is called the Rapid Diagnostic Test or RDT for short. The kids tend to be sicker and more prone to complications, such as cerebral malaria, respiratory distress, and anemia than the adults.

Adults will also catch malaria but tend to have milder symptoms since they have usually contracted malaria in the past and have some immunity to the infection. They complain of fever, headaches, and chills and may or may not have a palpable spleen. If a previously unexposed American catches malaria, they will be low sick like the kids.

Treatment consists of a three-day course of a combination drug call ACT. ACT will always contain Artesunate and a choice of several other antimalarial medications. ACT comes in different strengths depending on patient's age and weight. It seems to work effectively since I've not yet had any treated malaria patients return to the clinic.

I diagnosed a 10- year -old child with extrapulmonary TB this week. The girl had been having fever, night sweats, anorexia, and weight loss for several months. The poor child had been kept home by her parents for fear of exposing her to Ebola if she went to a hospital or clinic for care. It was a sad case of collateral damage due to Ebola in Liberia.

When I first saw the girl, it was hard to believe she was ten years old due to her cachexia. She had visible right cervical adenopathy that protruded laterally and down her neck in a matted chain. She also had a large soft nodule growing right out of her sternum. To make matters worse, she was terrified of white people or at least me. Her parents had to hold her down while she sobbed during my physical exam. There were no pulmonary symptoms or lung findings to speak of.

How do I know it was TB? I don't. There are no TB skin tests, x-rays, or biopsy services available in Fish Town. The little girl also saw a consulting Liberian PA who handles all the patients with HIV and other chronic infections, and he agreed with my diagnosis. The drugs used to treat children with extrapulmonary TB were not available in the clinic. They will have to be ordered from Monrovia and will take a couple of days to arrive. I gave her some nutritional supplements and Tylenol and hoped for the best. On a positive note, I did test her for HIV, and she was negative.

There is an upper respiratory infection making the rounds in Fish Town, and I have seen many patients, both young and old, with headaches, runny noses, dry cough, and general achiness. If they are generally healthy, I will give them some Tylenol and instructions to drink lots of fluids. We have no decongestants, and the only antihistamine we have is Benadryl. In some of the more frail and elderly patients, I will give a 5-day course of amoxicillin "just in case."

I had a patient today with a long history of asthma. He never smoked and had no occupational exposure that would have caused his pulmonary disease. He is a schoolteacher about my age and will begin teaching classes in one week. As soon as he entered my exam room, I could hear him wheezing. The only meds he had were Tylenol and cough syrup.

I had previously inquired about asthma medications available in the clinic. All they had was aminophylline tablets, a prehistoric medication more likely to make a patient sicker than well. I had scouted out several of the private pharmacies in town for additional medications. I had just purchased an aerosol albuterol inhaler I found a couple of days earlier.

When I pulled the inhaler out to give to him, he just about cried. He had used one in the distant past, and it had made a world of difference in his asthma. Since schools have been cancelled during the Ebola outbreak, he has not been paid for months and could not afford to buy any private medications. I added three days of prednisone for a boost, so he should be feeling pretty good in a day or so. Hopefully, next month he will be paid for his teaching, and he will be able to buy an inhaler himself. Albuterol inhalers cost $10 in Fish Town, a relative fortune in this economy. His was another case of collateral damage due to the Ebola epidemic. I ran into this patient a week later as I was taking a jungle walk. His breathing had returned to normal, and he was looking forward to returning to school.

I have also diagnosed a fair number of PID cases in younger women. PID is short for Pelvic Inflammatory Disease, an infection of the ovaries and fallopian tubes frequently caused by sexually transmitted bacteria such as gonorrhea. Even though provided with free condoms, men rarely use them and have multiple sex partners. I once made the mistake of asking a young woman how many times a week she has intercourse. "Two or three times a day," was her reply.

I definitely need to get my testosterone level checked when I return home.

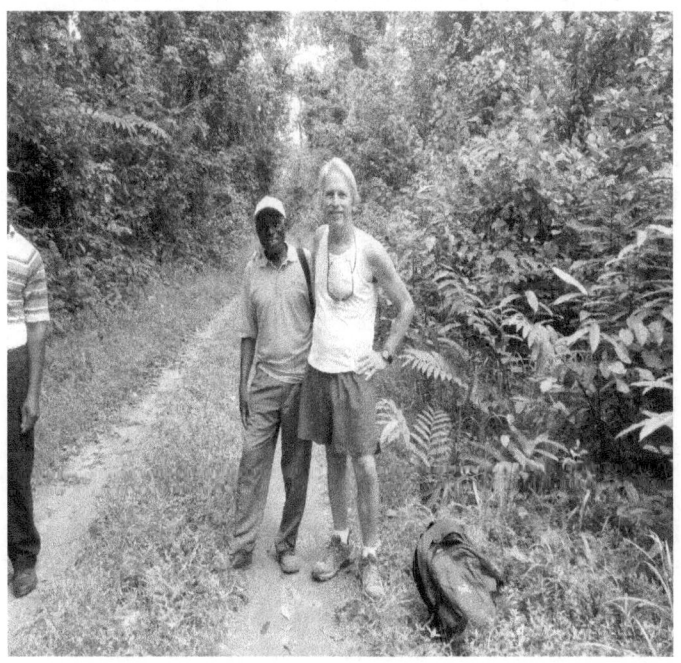

Schoolteacher that I treated for asthma

Fish Town 911

Monday is always one of the busiest days of the week at the Fish Town medical clinic. I arrived early to prepare for the onslaught of the sick and ailing. There was already a stack of charts on my desk of patients waiting to be seen. I have a Liberian nurse, Louise, who works with me to help translate Liberian English. She also helps me examine patients and write notes. She is battle hardened, rude, loud, and interrupts patients in midsentence. She gets them to quit talking about their family, the weather, or their feelings about the illness and cut to the chase. In short, she is the perfect nurse.

We take turns writing notes and examining patients. She does most of the interviewing and half the notes, and I write the prescriptions. We make good time, seeing about 6 to 8 patients an hour, but more charts are being added to our stack. It is the usual mix of young kids with malaria and respiratory illnesses along with adults complaining of fever, night sweats, and diffuse body aches.

The Liberian summer has arrived in force, and it gets up to 90 + degrees every afternoon with high humidity and rarely cools below 80 degrees at night. I observed that several of the patients who complained of fever and sweats were wearing jeans, undershirts, long sleeve shirts, and occasionally jackets. I wear the lightest pair of pants I own, always wear a short sleeve shirt, and I still sweat the entire day.

I examine the overheated, complaining patients, and other than an overabundant wardrobe, I find nothing wrong with them. I will occasionally order a malaria or typhoid test, but those are invariably negative. I sometimes politely suggest that perhaps they should consider wearing less clothing, but this recommendation is usually met with disbelief.

The average Liberian sense of cold and warmth is extremely skewed. Earlier in my journey, when the nights were cooler, I would awaken feeling energetic and comfortable in shorts and a T-shirt when the temperature was 70 degrees. I would go for walks outside and discover Liberians wearing insulated jackets or sweatshirts with the hoods over their heads. One night it got down to 60 degrees, and one of my Liberian roommates wore insulated underwear and a hoodie to bed and complained bitterly to his wife about how cold it was in Fish Town.
Back to the medical clinic.

About two hours into our schedule, a 12- year -old boy was brought in by his family for evaluation. He had been sick for months with fever, chills, weight loss, and generalized weakness. He had been seen multiple times at the clinic by medical providers for the same problems. He had been blindly treated with malaria meds, multiple antibiotics, and even worm medicine without improvement. Little lab testing had been done.

His exam revealed a listless young boy with jaundice, extreme cachexia, and a low- grade fever. His lungs were clear and his heart exam normal. He had massive enlargement of his spleen and liver. He had extreme muscle wasting and no fat on his body. I tested him for malaria, typhoid, and HIV, all of which were negative. He would die if the correct diagnosis was not made and treatment started soon.

I admitted the boy to the Fish Town Hospital, but his care there would not be much better. One of our team doctors has been working there, and she reported that the hospital had few medical supplies, no IV antibiotics, no x-ray, a pharmacy that was chronically short on medications, and a lab capable of doing only a few tests. There was only one government doctor working there, but he mainly did surgeries and was frequently out of town with his family in Monrovia. A physician assistant takes care of all the hospitalized patients.

At times I have been encouraged and elated in treating the simple, curable diseases in Liberia. However, there is also a certain amount of frustration that accompanies working in a medical environment with such severe deficiencies. At a modern medical facility the young boy would have been better evaluated and would have likely survived a treatable disease, but not in rural Liberia. The boy died 36 hours after admission. No cause of death was ever established.

On my way home from the clinic that afternoon, in the absolute worst heat and humidity of the day, I came across a young woman lying motionless in full sunlight on the side of the road. She did not respond to verbal questions nor move with physical stimuli, such as my foot nudging her body. She had shallow breathing, and I could see her neck pulsate, signifying she had a pulse.

Nearby vendors, selling pineapples and cell phone cards, had been watching me. I walked over and asked them how long the woman had been lying there. "About 15 or 20 minutes," was the reply.

I asked if anyone knew anything about her. "She has mental problems and drinks too much." Did she have any family nearby? "Yes, a brother."

I was joined by Kelsy and our head nurse, Demenia. We debated if we should call for an ambulance or take her in one of our vehicles. We decided to call an ambulance first. The brother appeared and confirmed that she had long term mental and alcohol problems. She had been found on the roads several times before and survived.

It was blazing hot. She lay on bare gravel, totally exposed to the sun. There was sweat glistening off her hot body, and her nostrils flared with mucus. We were on a steep hill and considered carrying her to a flat, shaded surface. But, even though there have been no Ebola patients reported in Fish Town for over 60 days, one needs to take pause before picking up an unknown collapsed patient with bare or even gloved hands. There are no second chances or Good Samaritan clauses in Ebola.

We stood patiently for 20 minutes and provided shade and poured cool water over her exposed skin. We heard several approaching combustible engines and hoped the ambulance was finally coming. But no, there were two hospital employees on motorcycles that were sent as a scouting team to see if an ambulance was really necessary.

They walked over, looked down at the girl, and recognized her. They confirmed the story of mental illness and alcohol abuse. I asked how and when they were going to move her to the hospital. "That is not necessary. She can just sleep it off."

After another 20 minutes of negotiation, the hospital employees finally agreed to roll her onto a blanket and carry her to a flat shaded area. I threw up my hands in disgust at that point and returned to the Fish Tank camp. I passed by later on in the day and saw that she was gone or at least out of sight. Out of sight, out of mind.

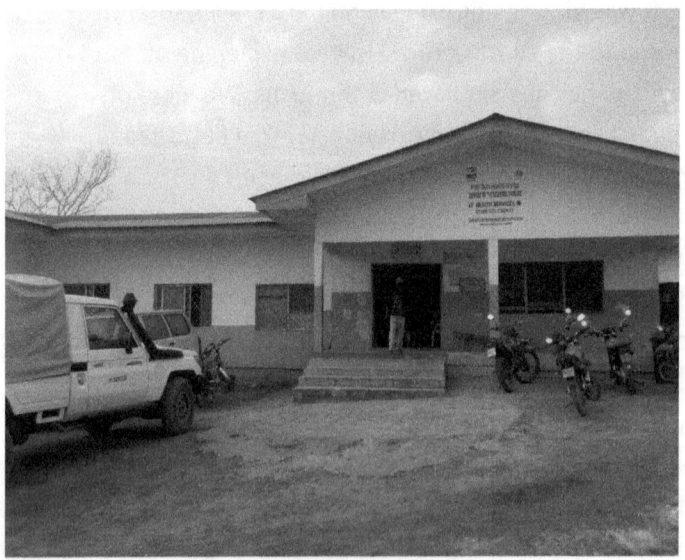

Fish Town medical clinic

Of Mice and Men

I have a new roommate. He is about 3 inches long with cute upright ears and goes by the name of Mickey. We have the same taste in crackers and cookies; although, he prefers to dine in the darkness of night.

I became aware of his presence when I reached for the crackers on my shelf and found the first two crackers with a hole gnawed in the middle. I have a slight overbite but not enough to cause this pattern of eating.

After that discovery, I started hanging my food in a bag near the ceiling. That was when I first spied my friend climbing up the inside wall of the tent. It was in the afternoon when I am usually out running errands, so we were both surprised to see each other. He noted my presence and made a quick retreat. I suspect he will return in the evening or early morning hours. I am at the point now where I don't mind sharing my food with others.

I see the skinny dogs that roam Fish Town, their noses to the ground constantly searching for food. The dogs are very skittish, and if you call or approach one, it will run away. Apparently, they have suffered much abuse at the hands of humans in the past. I have occasionally given a dog some leftover food while dining out, but that still did not buy me a tail wag or a soft pat on the head.

Cats are very rare in Fish Town and usually hang out in stores and bars where they are protected from the elements and predators. I saw a tuxedo cat that reminded me of an old cat we once owned. Tuxedo cats have distinctive black coats with a large white area on the chest.

Our tuxedo cat, Jack, was initially wild, hiding out in a ditch near our home. He would steal food from an outdoor bowl used by our domesticated cat. At first he would run when approached, but over time my eldest daughter, Ellen, was able to lure him closer and eventually pet him.

Jack was a wild beast with glaring yellow eyes and tolerated fools poorly. Our pampered cat, Katie, would routinely refuse any fresh fish or wild bird entrée. Jack would quietly creep up on me while I was cleaning fish or dove from an outdoors outing and steal a meal. Jack hated spending the night inside the house, preferring the primitive cathouse we had built outside.

The years of harsh outdoor living eventually caught up with Jack, and we found him lifeless one morning under his favorite tree. We buried him near that tree and placed a rock painted with his name on the grave. I still see that rock with the paint fading, and it brings back fond memories.

As my family can attest, I used to be a dedicated cat hater. I didn't care for their haughty attitude and refusal to follow commands. Now, in my later years, I have come to appreciate their free and independent spirit. While I still prefer a dog as a pet, I also enjoy the presence of a cat in my life, for the softness of their fur and the vibration of their purring when they lie in my lap. I have turned into a softie.

Our one surviving cat is Katie, the "Cancer Cat." She is now over 20 years old (>100 years in cat years) and will probably outlive me. We adopted her as a kitten when my youngest daughter, Amy, was just 4 years old.

We call Katie the "Cancer Cat" because we adopted her when Amy was just starting treatment for cancer on her tongue. During a nine-month span, Amy first underwent surgery on her tongue, followed by radiation, and then six months of chemotherapy. Amy lost all of her hair and wasted down to 40 pounds. Through it all Amy would carry Katie around with her, often by the neck. But Katie never bit and rarely scratched Amy despite all the rough handling. The chemo caused low white blood cell and platelet counts, making Amy susceptible to infections and bleeding. I believe Katie warded off trauma and infections with her very presence.

This past summer Amy married a true gentleman, Max Cathcart. Twenty years ago I thought I had a better chance of burying Amy than marrying her off. My life has been full of miracles.

Katie lives in our garage now. She treats the litter box like she is playing horseshoes with more misses than hits. She has lost many of her teeth and can only eat soft food. Before leaving for Africa, I was her primary caretaker, cleaning up her litter box misses, and experimenting with different flavors of high dollar canned cat food.

If it's a nice day, Katie will still venture out onto our driveway to enjoy a little sunshine. She plays "chicken" when we pull into our garage by slowly parading in front of our vehicle as we patiently wait for her to pass. She has earned my respect, and I will miss her when she's gone.

Insect Invasion!

With the arrival of the Liberian summer, there has been a series of different insects swarming around our lights, crawling into our tents and beds, and surprising us in the showers and bathrooms. Initially, small black flies appeared to be undergoing their annual mating ritual around our lights. They would fill the sky, coupling in midair, with their tiny wings whirling, then fall to the ground and die. In the morning there would be piles of their dead bodies covering the floors of our dining areas and bathrooms. I hope it was good for them.

The small fly love festival lasted one week and was soon followed by giant rhinoceros beetles. These are impressive specimens, fully worthy of their name. The ones here in Liberia are about the size of your palm and have pinchers that will give you pause. One night we found two rhinoceros beetles locked in combat. We put them on a table and placed bets on which beetle would triumph. Yes, we are that desperate for entertainment in the Fish Tank.

Since then the common housefly has emerged and is by far the most annoying insect we have encountered. They get into our tents in the day and night and proceed to torture us by landing on our necks, shoulders, legs, arms, and anywhere else where we can't quickly slap them away. We have requested fly swatters, but that plea fell on deaf ears. Having a fan blow full blast will usually keep them off of you. Unfortunately, the generators that power the fans only run three hours in the afternoon and the flies are the worst in the morning and latter part of the day.

Small sugar ants have also moved into our tents and buildings. They have a remarkable sense of smell and taste. They can find the tiniest amount of sugar or food left on a spoon, cup, or shelf. I found long strands of the ants marching back and forth from a closed bucket I previously thought impregnable. I took the lid off to discover a small opened package of cookies swarming with the ants...another source of protein I can add to my diet.

Army ants are present here in Liberia, but fortunately, live mostly in the jungle. They are good sized, about an inch in length, and black in color. On my hikes, I have walked past thick strands of army ants stretched across the road when a particularly good food item has been discovered. One time I accidently stepped on a line of army ants and was rewarded with several nasty bites on my ankle. In the future, I will make a wide detour if I meet them.

There are some beautiful moths here. They are huge in size, filling your entire hand. I have seen bright yellow moths, brown textured moths with black dots on the wings that look like eyes, and one orange moth with what appears to be a snakehead on the tip of each wing. I usually try to get a picture if I can. When I was staying at the Worst 8 Motel, I found a beautiful yellow moth in the lobby one morning and pointed it out to an employee. He immediately smashed it with his foot and laughed heartily. So much for moth appreciation in Liberia.

A type of locust has also made an appearance in the last week. They are about three inches long with brown wings and resemble the roach from hell that greets you in the middle of the night in your Texas kitchen. They, too, are making their annual migration and will die in your tents and buildings for your discovery.

Wasps are always a threat in hot climates. You will be glad to know that Liberia has a very healthy population of black, red, and yellow wasps that are ready to provide venom to those unwary souls who dare to cross them. They particularly like to hang out in the bathrooms and showers where you are most exposed and vulnerable. Part of my shower selection process includes a survey for stinging and biting insects. Who says I don't have a mission here?

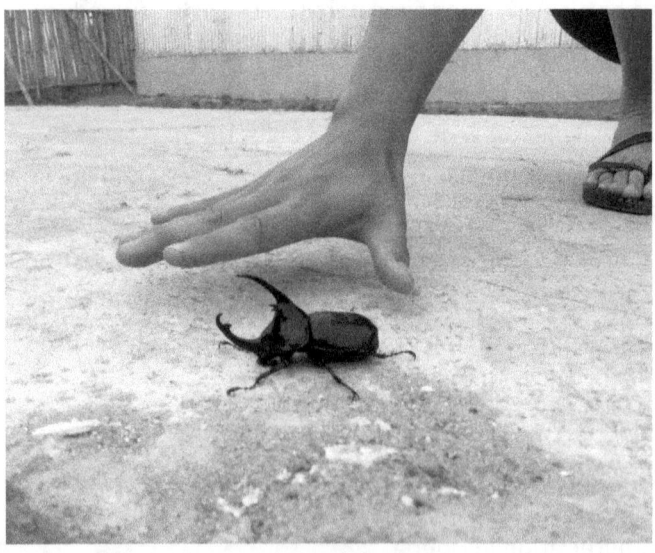

Rhinoceros beetle in Liberia

The Sex Lives of Ebola Medical Workers

Use your imagination.

We did.

The end.

Dr. Joe of Fish Town

Snake Hunt

Mark, Kelsy, and Jonathan go for frequent walks into the jungle on the surrounding roads. On one of their recent outings, they reported coming upon a large dead snake that stretched clear across the single-lane road.

I asked for more details about the monster snake. "It had a lump in its belly that was probably a rat or small mammal."

"What else?" I asked.

"It was black and it was dead."

No mention of head shape, fangs, or skin pattern. No photos were taken. Clearly this would require further investigation on my part.

Early the next morning, I stuffed a liter of water and a camera into my backpack and started down the road. As I left the outskirts of Fish Town, I passed by isolated houses with packs of children waving wildly at me. I waved back, but the novelty has definitely faded. I passed several women carrying pineapples and other goods into town for sale in the market. I also passed many men and boys with large machetes. I gave them an extra big smile and hello for obvious self-preservation reasons.

The road was hilly and eroded as I pushed deeper into the jungle. It narrowed to just a single lane that could barely contain a vehicle. I came upon a large mud hole taking up the center of the road. When I tried to walk along the right perimeter, I heard a loud hissing sound and saw the grass moving a few feet away from me. I took a quick step to the other side, but saw and heard nothing else from the grass.

I crossed several creeks with wooden, makeshift bridges that required tightrope like steps. I eventually came to a sizeable river with a recently built concrete bridge spanning it. I looked over the railing at what should have been the ultimate snake habitat, but saw none. The giant, dead snake described by my teammates was no more. What kind of snake hunt was this?

I had been walking for an hour and a half, and it was time to turn around. As I returned home, I passed three young men carrying cane poles with black braided line and small hooks. It was obvious what they were up to.

I stopped and asked them about the fishing here in River Gee County. They were headed towards the big river I just visited. They reported catching many small fish and an occasional larger catfish using worms for bait. In the global language of all fishermen, I wished them good luck in their endeavors.

On the return trip to Fish Town, I caught a glimpse of a sizeable snake as it slithered across the road ahead of me and disappeared into the jungle. I did not pursue the snake into the jungle. Although I have an unhealthy interest in snakes, I am not insane.

Near the conclusion of my walk, I took a side road up to the top of the highest hill in Fish Town. I was curious about a partially completed concrete structure visible from our camp. I passed a nearby house, and a couple of kids ran out to play "Touch the White Man." I am also growing tired of being touched by snotty nosed kids.

The concrete structure at the top of the hill was either

going to be a very large home or guest house. There were many small rooms on the perimeter and a couple of larger rooms in the interior. Weeds had grown up around and inside the stagnant structure. I pulled myself up and over the outer wall to get a better view.

From this overlook, our camp was plainly visible with its large white storehouse at the top and multiple, large, green tents cascading down the hillside. Downtown Fish Town sits behind our camp and was most notable for the clouds of red dust that drifted up from the main road due to the constant motorcycle and vehicular traffic.

I descended the hill and returned to our camp very tired, sweaty, and dirty. I took a cold shower, put on running shorts, and tried to take a nap. The constant chatter of the workers and other camp noises kept me from actually sleeping.

At dinner that evening Jonathan and Kelsy told me that they took the same walk later that afternoon and saw not one, but two snakes, one of which was neatly cut up into multiple pieces by a machete. We now call the road "The Snake Walk" to distinguish it from other hikes we take. I will try to walk it again next week, and maybe I will get lucky.

The 7- foot Cobra

I returned from work today after 1 p.m. and was immediately surrounded by my fellow coworkers and snake enthusiasts. A large black snake was seen on my patio earlier this afternoon. It slithered down a hole before anyone could take a picture or kill it. My companions told me the snake was coming straight for my tent because of all my snake shirts and coffee cups.

I was bitterly disappointed at this missed snake encounter and scouted the area off my patio where the snake was last sighted. The snake disappeared near a bamboo and chain link fence. The area has much grass and bushes in which to hide and stalk prey. It was perfect snake habitat.

There were several African men who were even more interested in the snake than me. Once a snake has been sighted in our campground, something must be done to remove the potential threat of a lethal snakebite. The African snakes are not to be trivialized. Their venom can kill a man in minutes. The nearest antivenom is hundreds of miles and days away from Fish Town.

I was trying to write some stories when thick smoke started pouring into the entrance of my tent. A couple of men had gone outside the perimeter fence and were burning a tire to smoke the snake out of its hole. I considered this activity as more of a fire hazard than a good way to kill a snake. I was about to be schooled in African Snake Hunting 101.

I returned to my tent and twenty minutes passed with

the smelly black smoke billowing up and into our tents. Several men stood around with shovels and long bamboo poles intently watching the hole where the snake disappeared.

Suddenly, there was shouting and screaming coming from the snake watch area and I raced outside my tent. I immediately saw one of the biggest snakes I have ever seen out of captivity. It was sinister black, at least 6 feet long, and slithered with its head up in the air. The snake escaped from its hole and was now isolated on the bare gravel ground that was my back yard.

The snake hunters were absolutely fearless. Six men attempted to beat the snake with long bamboo poles, shovels, and pieces of lumbar. The snake was surrounded and could not escape. It then rose up at least three feet in the air and struck at the poles and boards. Someone was finally able to deliver a solid blow to the snake's head and it fell to the ground where multiple blows were delivered. The huge snake writhed on the ground for several more minutes as additional blows were delivered. A shovel was used to finally crush its head.

The snake was measured and held up for inspection. A crowd of more than 50 people was drawn into the excitement. The snake was over 7 feet long and was identified as a cobra, one of the most lethal and aggressive of all African snakes. Many photos were taken, and one man even held it up by the tail. The snake was eventually taken to a nearby neighbor's house and cooked for dinner.

I wanted to see one of these lethal African snakes, and I definitely had an up close experience. I think I will back off on my snake hunts for the time being.

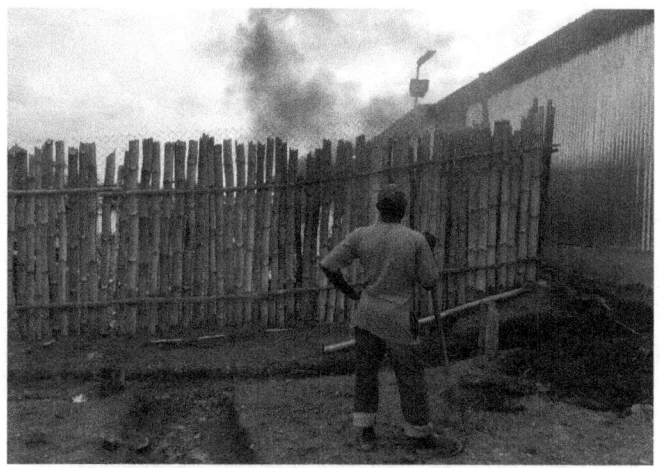

Smoking a snake out of its hole.

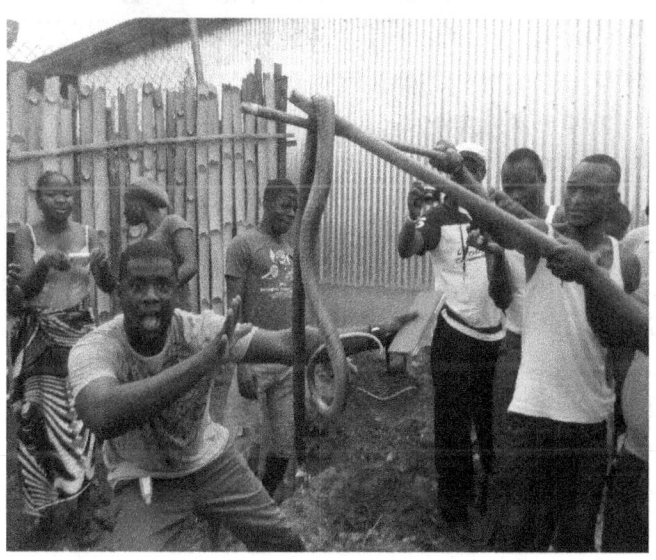

Snake on a Stick

Dr. Joe Spann

And Sometimes You Just Run Out of Piss

Dear Family and Friends,

It has been a running joke among my medical coworkers in Liberia that our efforts here are like pissing in an ocean of human misery. It's just not going to make a difference. But I don't buy it. I believe if you can just help that one patient to get better or recover, then you have made a big difference in that person's life.

I have been going to the Fish Town medical clinic for three weeks now, seeing anywhere from 100 to 150 patients a week. My efforts have been appreciated by the locals who have spread the word that a "White Man with good medicine" is in town.

I have started seeing many local politicians and their families, police officers, tribal leaders, clinic and hospital employees, and various other local dignitaries. While it has been rewarding and flattering, I woke up the other morning and thought, "I don't want to go to work today."

I got up anyway, dressed, and started the one- mile walk to the medical clinic. The usual groups of small children waved to me calling out, "Hello White Man!" As I walked along the dusty gravel roads, I dodged the murderous motorcycles while threading my way through the piles of discarded cans and plastic bags that littered the ground.

I entered the Fish Town medical clinic and saw the halls already full of crying babies, restless young children, pregnant women, and older adults. And I thought to myself, "I hate this place. I want to go home." And so I am.

As part of my employment contract with ARC, I am allowed an early termination with 30 days' notice. I would stay if I was actively treating Ebola patients, but there are no Ebola patients in River Gee County, Liberia. The medical work I have been performing here has been voluntary and supplements the Liberian government employees. It is helpful but not essential.

I have made some good friends and lasting memories while in Liberia, but it is time for me to go home. I have another family that needs me.

As Kelsy so wisely said, "Sometimes you just run out of piss."

See you soon.

Love,

Joe

Last Night in Fish Town

I am heading home. But before I can leave, I must say goodbye to my teammates who have been my friends and family for the past 80 days. I found out Friday afternoon that my departing flight would be Monday night out of Monrovia. I will need to leave the next morning by vehicle to make the flight.

I told my closest teammates one at a time during the day. They were happy that I was going home but said they will miss me. It has been a rough journey together, and rather than hate each other, we have bonded tightly. I feel like a deserter.

We gathered for drinks at sunset on my patio. I pulled out all my leftover liquor bottles, food, medications, batteries, and other survival supplies that I will no longer need. I placed them in a large open box and offered them up for anyone dropping by. The liquor bottles went quickly, not unexpected with this crowd. The cookies and canned peaches followed. My suture materials were perused and deemed better quality than what exists at the local medical clinic and hospital. Eventually, as I had hoped, the box was empty.

Jonathan and Mark dropped by my tent afterwards and had a quick toast. We recalled ten weeks ago in Minneapolis when we went out for dinner the night before leaving for Liberia. We remembered the exact drinks and food we ordered. We made a toast that night to each other and our "great adventure." At the time, we each thought one of us was going to die of Ebola in Liberia. Guess we will have to skip the tragic ending.

Our cooks, Reginal and Jebbeh, wanted to take me downtown one last time for drinking and dancing. I knew this would mostly involve me buying the drinks and them drinking and dancing, but tonight I did not care. The cooks are the hardest working people in the Fish Tank and deserve some fun.

I left the Fish Tank with no less than three of the cooks in tow. They were dressed to kill and looked dangerous with short skirts and tight tops. We walked in the dark up and down steep gravel hills with lots of ruts to trip us up. I had a few drinks by then, but the cooks held both of my hands so I would not fall.

We arrived at the bar where the music was blasting, and immediately all the young men were hitting on the girls. But tonight the girls were all mine. They brushed off would be suitors, and we began the drinking. I ordered a single beer for myself, but the girls were taking doubles. After a few rounds they took turns dancing with the old white man. I have been an ardent observer of the Liberian dance style that resembles wild animals mating and attempted to duplicate it. I was absolutely no good at the dancing, but I admit it did have its finer points. I doubt I will be performing it at my hometown dancehall, the Broken Spoke, anytime soon.

This went on until almost midnight when Brendon, our Irish engineer, came to rescue me. No doubt the cooks would party on until the wee hours of the morning, but I had a long day's worth of travel ahead. Brendon gently led me away, but not before Reginal caught me, swore eternal love to me and asked, "Can I have another $20 Dr. Joe?"

I made it home safely with Brendon's assistance, and there was a large cardboard sign on our bulletin board with "Goodbye Dr. Joe. We will miss you, Your Fish Tank Family." I felt guilty once more for leaving early, but it is too late now to turn back. Besides, I have another family I need to take care of, and they are thousands of miles away.

Goodbye my Fish Town friends and family.

Dr. Joe

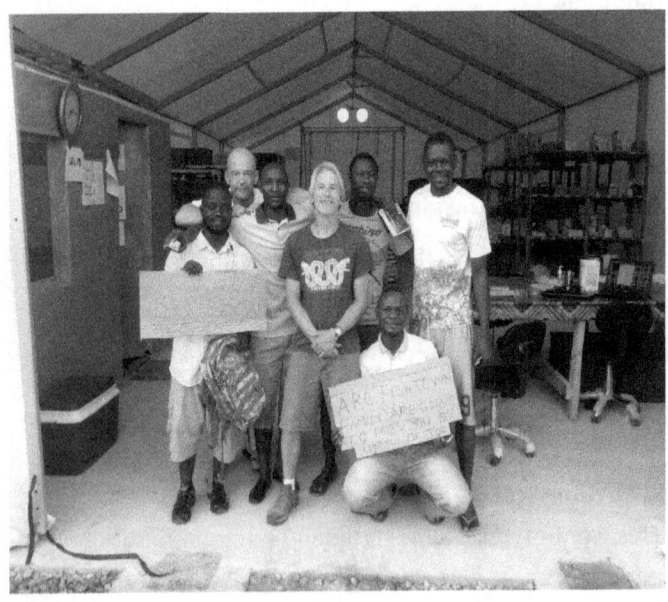

Dr. Joe and friends

Road Back to Monrovia

In the morning, after a few more sad farewells to my teammates, I climbed aboard our 4 -wheel drive Ford pickup. It was the same one I arrived in and the one used for my infamous trip to Harper. It is a badass truck and today was being driven by Jojo, a badass in his own right. He has family back in Monrovia, and he drove like a horse racing back to the stable after a trail ride. We also had Richardson, our IT guy, riding with us. And the biggest honor of all….the great Cece of Cece's Bar fame would be with us!

Cece grew up in Monrovia and started the bar in Fish Town with the help of her brother. She liked to visit Monrovia four to five times a year for a week or so and stock up on supplies she could not find in Fish Town.

We got going about 9 am, which was an early start for Liberians. I loaded my suitcases into the bed of the pickup and covered them with trash bags in an attempt to keep the eternal red dust off. I let Richardson ride shotgun because he was a bigger fellow than me and I wished to chat with Cece on the drive. Traditionally, the white people ride up front, but I have been changing that norm whenever possible.

We bumped along on the typical Liberian road for about an hour, and Cece was unusually quiet. Suddenly, she was throwing up into a paper bag that she had prophetically brought along. It is of significance that on both road trips to and from Fish Town there has been a Liberian throwing up in the back seat. These roads will take the most tested individuals down. I medicated her with some oral Phenergan and periactin in an attempt to help her nausea, but all it did was make her sleepy.

We got a flat tire about half way through the day, so we all piled out of the truck. Jojo tried to lower the spare tire down from under the truck but had trouble getting the long handle wrench to fit into the correct hole. I slid under the tilting truck to manually place the wrench head into the hole. I came out covered in red dust but didn't care. I needed to get home and this truck had to get me there.

The spare tire was lowered, but now the metal holding device wouldn't let loose. Once again, I slithered under the truck and physically removed the restraining metal piece from the tire. Another layer of red dirt was added to my clothing. After that the flat tire was quickly removed and replaced with the spare. The flat tire was shredded and could not be repaired. A replacement tire in Ganta City would cost $300 . We decided to drive the rest of the way to Monrovia with no spare. Wish us luck.

We made it to Ganta City and checked into the Alvino Hotel, the same fine establishment where Jonathan and I shared a room on the way to Fish Town nearly two months earlier. While it was a decidedly crash course in getting to know my teammates, it did bring back fond memories.

I was upgraded to the Chico VIP suite which, for $15 extra, had a living room, small kitchen, king bed, AC, TV, electricity, private bathroom with shower, and running cold water. I have reserved the Chico suite for Jonathan and me for our reunion tour in 2020.

I went out for dinner with Jojo, Richardson, and Cece at a fine nearby restaurant. I had the pepper soup with cow meat, and it was pretty good. This was followed by a few beers at a local disco and bar where some young women were dancing in unison to recorded music. The Liberian women were looking better and better every day to my celibate eyes. I am leaving just in time.

I returned to my hotel room and tried watching some TV. There was BBC, but who can ever understand what the British are saying? There was nothing nearly as entertaining as the daily Fish Tank reality show I had been living in for the past two months.

The next morning was a Sunday, and we got an early start, skipping my requisite hot tea and energy drink since all the stores were closed. Surprisingly, the roads improved as we cruised along, and before long we were speeding along on brand new pavement with fresh paint marking the lanes!

Apparently, there was a national road improvement project planned before the Ebola epidemic. It was put on hold for many months, but was now starting up. It was a remarkable sight to witness such a game changing event for a country that had been down on its luck for many years. With good roads, produce and products can be rapidly transported throughout the nation and to the world. This will generate jobs and income for the Liberian people. There is a definite wisp of hope in the air for Liberia.

Large stretches of highway had been graded but were still dirt and gravel. Even so, it was a vast improvement from the previous road. We passed roadside stands manned by locals, and we stopped at one to pick up some food items and charcoal. There is a type of large insect larva that is harvested from the local trees and sold alive and wiggling in narrow plastic bags. They are apparently quite delicious when cooked and prepared properly. I examined the fat, wiggling, yellow larvae and decided to take their word for how good they taste.

We made it to Monrovia before noon and dropped Cece off. She would be picked up by her brother. I gave her a hug and promised to return to Fish Town someday. We drove to a nearby creek and stopped. There were several young men and boys who competed for the job of washing our truck. After a brief negotiation, a couple of boys were selected. We stood on the side of the road as our truck was washed.

I looked around at the outlying suburb of Monrovia and was thankful that I did not spend my entire trip there. Monrovia has a lot of advantages that a big city can provide, but it also has a huge population packed into a small area. It is overwhelming at times with the noise, crowding, and pollution. At least in Fish Town I was able to get to know my neighbors quite well and enjoy the remoteness of the nearby jungle.

We dropped Richardson off at his house and drove over to Jojo's newly built home. Jojo was quite proud of his home, and he should be. It sat well off the noisy road, on a hillside, with a big yard and expansive view. His wife had prepared lunch for us and we sat outside at a table under a shade tree to eat.

The lunch was delicious with a fresh seafood sauce served over rice. My hands got totally messy while attempting to extract every ounce of meat from the shellfish. Fortunately, his wife brought out a washcloth and bowl of warm water in anticipation of my messy ways.

Afterwards I was driven to the original apartment where I started my adventure in Liberia nearly three months earlier. I was given the master suite since it happened to be vacant that night. Walter was there along with a new roommate, Lisa, who was involved in international public health. I spent the afternoon doing laundry and attempting to remove the diesel smell from my suitcases, which were soaked during the drive from Fish Town.

That night, Walter, Lisa, and I did some tequila shots from the last of the Patron I purchased months before. We went out to dinner at Fuzion, an upscale restaurant and bar not far from our apartment. We sat outside on an open balcony, and I ordered a Smokey Joe to appease Walter who will forever associate that drink with me. Unfortunately, they were out of the tiny umbrellas that usually garnish the drink, and it just did not taste the same. I had a great dinner of fresh fish and mango sauce and enjoyed a reflective conversation with Walter and Lisa.

Tomorrow will be my last day in Liberia, and I have much to do in preparation for departure. Cramming all my clothes, equipment, and souvenirs into my suitcases will be difficult. Putting all the emotions and experiences of the past three months into my memory will be impossible, but I will try.

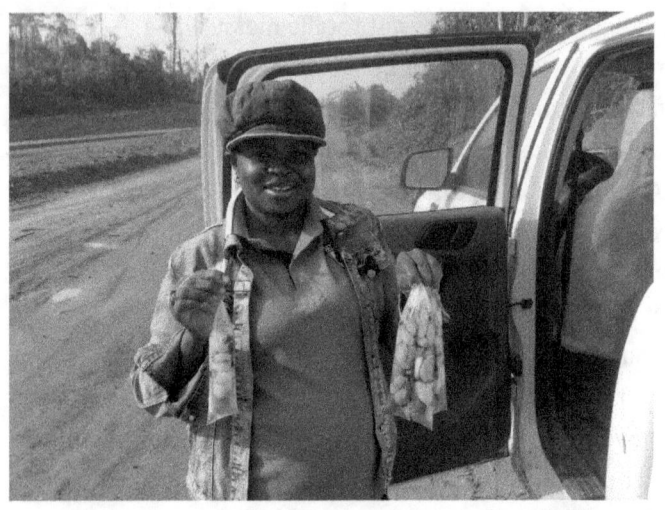

Cece with some fresh larvae

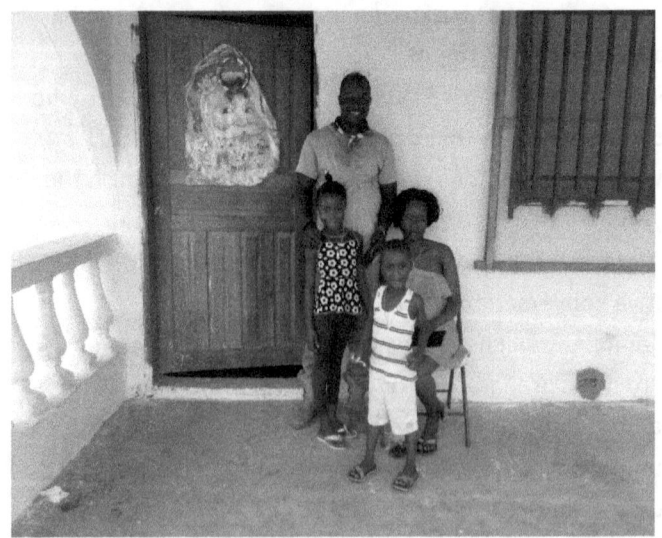

Jojo and family

Last Day in Liberia

My flight from Monrovia to Brussels is at 9:30 p.m. I spent my final day in Liberia shopping for last minute souvenirs. I bought another suitcase to transport all the different items I have purchased while traveling here. Most of them I will probably not care about in a few months, but some I will treasure forever. How many folks have scrub shirts made of way cool African fabric?

I also met Rose, the midwife from Fish Town, for lunch at the swanky Mamba Point Hotel. She had moved to Monrovia the week before to start classes at the university. Her dream is to become an Ob-Gyn doctor and practice in Liberia.

We sat outside on a patio that overlooked the beach and ocean. The menu was global cuisine, including sushi, Italian, American, and Lebanese items. Rose was disappointed to find no African food on the menu. We asked the waiter if there was African food available, and he brought us a separate menu with national food listed. I kidded Rose that while I was in Fish Town all I ever ate was African food, and now she wouldn't eat one meal of American food with me. Rose decided that she would try American food to appease me, but for some reason ordered sushi and lasagna. I didn't bother to correct her and ordered a salad and some fish for myself.

When the sushi arrived at our table, Rose examined it carefully. She had never before eaten sushi but identified rice in the rolls and tried one. She chewed it carefully, waiting to see what it would taste like. She liked it! I pointed to the ginger on the side, and Rose speared a forkful to put in her mouth all at once. I interceded and recommend trying one slice at a time. She put one piece in her mouth for a short while then spit it out. Not a ginger fan.

The lasagna arrived steaming hot, and it was a huge piece. Rose tried a few bites but did not care for it. I ended up packing the lasagna as a take-out item to eat later on my departure plane.

We shopped for a while on the beachfront, purchasing a couple of purses for my girls back home and a pair of oven mitts made out of African fabric. I love practical stuff that also looks cool.

We walked the beach where I got my feet gloriously wet and sandy one last time. The waves were large, so I played chicken with the surf. Rose seemed to enjoy me getting wet but wouldn't get near the water herself.

We returned to the street and called a driver to pick us up. It was rush hour in Monrovia, and we slowly inched our way home through the crowded, noisy streets. Pedestrians, cabs, motorcycles, and vehicles fought for every advantage. We finally broke out of the traffic and got close to the apartment where I could pick up my luggage and head for the airport.

Rose got out about a mile from my destination and said goodbye. I have promised to send her some money from time to time to help with her education and training. She is the future hope for Liberia if it is ever to have enough doctors to care for the nation's population. My work here may have no sustainability, but perhaps by supporting Rose, my brief presence here will last for many years to come.

I suspect most readers will think that Rose and I have a romance going on. And I guess we do. I love her strength, intelligence, and drive to improve her life and those of her fellow Liberians. She has never asked me for money. She is engaged but has no wedding date set. On this final goodbye she gives me a kiss on the cheek, the only kiss I ever received from her. No lip kissing here. After all, this is Ebola country.

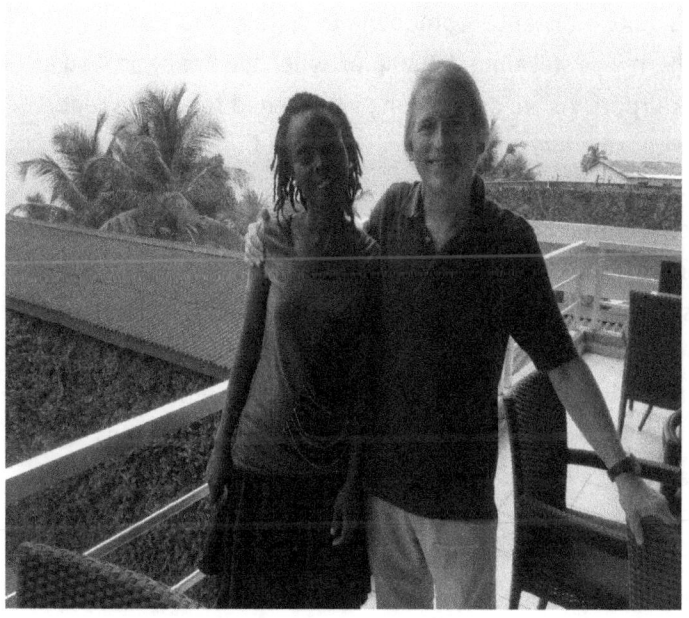

Rose and me at the Mamba Point Hotel

The Long Road Home: Part 1

My flight from Monrovia to Brussels was scheduled for 9:30 p.m. My driver was Alfred who I knew well from my travels to Fish Town and Harper. He likes to drive fast, passing on hills and curves, darting in and out between cars, and honking the horn constantly; in short, my kind of Liberian driver. We were accompanied by Stephanie, an ARC assistant, who would help me navigate the Monrovia airport and boarding process.

We left at 6 p.m. since it was rush hour, and the airport was quite a distance from town. Despite Alfred's driving skills, it was still almost 7:30 p.m. when we finally arrived at the airport. As we drove along we listened to a radio report announcing five new Ebola cases in a suburb of Monrovia. Sometimes I think fighting Ebola is like "Whack a Mole". A cluster of cases will pop up in one area of Liberia to be contained, only to have another cluster of cases appear elsewhere in another week or so. It was disheartening to know that as I left Liberia, the Ebola virus continued to survive despite every healthcare provider's best efforts.

Before we entered the Monrovia Airport grounds Stephanie climbed into the back of the SUV to hide amongst my luggage. Since the arrival of the Ebola epidemic, the airport only allows the passenger and one other person to enter the terminal. Alfred and I had our temperatures taken through the SUV windows before we could enter the parking area. After we parked, Stephanie climbed out of the back, and we approached the terminal entrance.

On the stairs leading into the terminal, I had my temperature taken again. I completed an extensive questionnaire on where I had been, where I was going, passport number, and all my contact information. Stephanie and Alfred were forced to stay outside, but they were able to monitor my progress in the airport through a large outside door.

They arranged for an airport porter to assist me with my three large bags. We made our way through a narrow passageway packed with travelers and, once more, my temperature was taken before I could enter the terminal building proper. It was hot and humid, and all my clothes were soaked in sweat. I worried that my temperature was going to read too high, and I wouldn't be able to ever go home.

I finally made it up to the Brussels Airline ticket desk. They asked for the usual ID and ticket information, but I became concerned when they asked if my final destination was Houston. Initially, my sponsoring organization had made airline reservations for me to go to Houston, mixing me up with Terry, our engineer and another Texas white guy.

I informed them of the mistake a couple of days prior to my departure, and they reassured me that the reservation had been corrected to show Austin as my final destination. The airline clerk did another search in her computer, found the correct ticket reservation, and all was well.

I had purchased another suitcase to bring all my souvenirs home, bumping my total up to 3 bags, one more than is customarily allowed. It will cost me $200 in cash for the extra bag. Fortunately, I knew this in advance and had over $500 on me. But it was not that simple. I had to leave my bags at the desk and go outside the terminal to the airline's office to pay the $200.

An airline employee guided me through the crowds to the terminal exit and pointed to the airline office about 100 feet away. A Liberian appeared at my side and offered to accompany me to the office, and I accepted. I would accept any and all help at this point. We walked across the gravel lot, and I entered the office while he waited outside. Inside there were forms to be completed and signed. After I paid the $200, I was given a receipt that I was to return to the ticket agents. My guide, who was waiting for me as I exited the office, led me back to the terminal entrance where I had to explain to the security guard and nurse that I had already been through this line once and was just trying to return to the ticket desk inside. They eyed me suspiciously, but after my guide confirmed my story, I was allowed to skip the repeat temperature and questionnaire and return to the ticket desk. I tipped my guide $1 and stepped on in. My receipt for the extra bag was accepted, and I was issued my flight tickets home.

Next, my baggage was searched by airport security before being loaded on the plane. My assistant lifted each heavy bag onto the table and security dug through my dirty laundry and gear. I was a little worried one of my bags would be rejected because it got soaked in diesel fuel during the ride from Fish Town to Monrovia. It still smelled of diesel fuel, despite my best efforts to scrub it out with dishwashing liquid the day before. The diesel smell did not seem to bother the security guard and neither did the two machetes that I impulsively purchased on my last day in Fish Town. Just in case.

I took a seat in the waiting room with about 100 other travelers. I saw more white people than I had seen in the past three months. The majority of the travelers were departing healthcare workers who were returning to their respective countries. Most of the travelers were sitting quietly by themselves or with another teammate. The healthcare workers had a tired appearance and were not interested in making conversation with anyone. They were like me. They just wanted to go home.

There was a gift shop off the waiting room with overpriced Liberia souvenirs. I considered an "I Love Liberia" T-shirt, but it was $20 and of poor quality. Ebola boom economy at work again.

The boarding began, and I found my way to a window seat with an empty seat next to me. The plane was only about half full and provided lots of room for the exhausted healthcare workers to stretch out and sleep. But first a hot meal was served consisting of Brie cheese, fresh bread, real butter, cold macaroni salad, and the best cow meat ever. I washed it down with complimentary wine, and I was in heaven.

I was seated close to several Chinese Ebola workers. The Chinese ETU in Monrovia is the only ETU in Liberia that is air-conditioned. Sissies.

I dozed off and on in the darkness of the cabin during our six- hour flight. My thoughts were now focused on friends and family I would see on my return. It had been over 10 weeks since I left for Liberia, the longest separation ever from my wife. June is the smartest, most loving, patient woman I have ever known, and I feel blessed to have her as my wife. Sometimes you have to leave somebody to realize how important he or she is in your life.

Six hours passed quickly. The lights went on in the cabin, and the stewardesses pushed carts down the aisles, passing out coffee, tea, and a cold breakfast. As we neared Brussels, I gazed out the window and was amazed to see so many lights on the ground. I have taken for granted how important such things as electricity and other public utilities are for a country and its development. Without electricity, businesses cannot function efficiently, products cannot be made in quantity, and the darkness of night prohibits meaningful work for half the day. Liberia's scant electricity is primarily provided by individual generators that usually run just part of the day due to the high cost of fuel. I did pass through one part of the country where the electricity was supplied by a hydroelectric dam, but that was the exception rather than the norm.

We landed softly in Brussels and filed off the airplane, once more having our temperatures taken. Belgium and most Western European countries do not require quarantine for returning Ebola workers. I seriously considered spending my first 21 days in Western Europe but then became too homesick, and the thought of spending another three weeks living out of a suitcase was not appealing.

Walking through the Brussels airport, I passed a large exhibit honoring Flanders Fields, a very small part of Belgium, where some of the fiercest and deadliest battles raged during WWI. With an estimated loss (on both sides) of over 400,000 men, the battles in Flanders Fields rank among the deadliest confrontations of the war.

Passing the exhibit, I recalled the poem "In Flanders Fields", which I was required to memorize while in grade school in Tulsa, Oklahoma.

"In Flanders fields the poppies blow

Between the crosses, row on row"

I looked up, and there were hundreds of artificial red poppies hanging from the ceiling.

"In Flanders Fields" was written by Lt. Colonel John McCrae, a doctor, during his service in the Canadian Army in 1915. He had just lost a friend, killed in action the day before. He was sitting on the step of an army ambulance and saw the beds of blood-red poppies growing between the graves in the burial ground. McCrae worked on his poem for several months before submitting it to the literary magazine *Spectator* in London where it was promptly rejected. It was later published anonymously in *Punch*, the weekly British satirical magazine.

"In Flanders Fields" became the most popular poem of that time, but McCrae would not live to see his legacy confirmed. He died of meningitis in 1918. Because of his poem, the poppy became an international symbol of remembrance of soldiers killed in WWI.

I had a six hour layover in Brussels before my flight to Washington, D.C., only one of four airports in the United

States designated as entry points for returning West African Ebola medical workers. I spent my time writing and drinking lots of caffeinated beverages. I also bought some Belgian chocolates for my family and friends. Belgian chocolate is reportedly the best in the world. I know it costs that much.

The flight from Brussels to Washington, D.C. was full, and I ended up in a dreaded middle seat for the 8- hour flight. The fellow to the right of me was generously proportioned and immediately claimed the armrest between us and a couple of inches beyond. I attempted to politely apply pressure to his invasive elbow, but he didn't budge. I was in for a long flight.

The lady seated to my left was a returning American-Liberian. She worked for the NIH and was working on the Ebola vaccine trials. We had a prolonged conversation about Ebola and Liberia in general. She thanked me for going to Liberia in the fight against Ebola. I don't believe I deserve much credit for fighting Ebola since I saw just a handful of patients in Bong County during my training. I am not so much an Ebola fighter as I am an Ebola soldier. I left my home, trained for battle, but saw little action. The men and women who arrived and served earlier in the Ebola epidemic are the true Ebola fighters and heroes.

The Long Road Home: Part 2

When we last left off, I was flying from Brussels to Washington, D.C. in the middle seat squeezed between an oversized gentleman and a woman from the NIH. It was an 8-hour flight, but the time passed quickly while I practiced my breath holding skills.

We landed at Washington Dulles Airport and filed off the airplane. It was 2:40 pm, with seemingly plenty of time before my 5:00 pm flight to Austin. I was mixed with all the other passengers as I entered the US Immigration checkpoint. I waited for 20 minutes in a line with a coughing child who was more of an infectious risk than me. When I finally took my turn with the Immigration agent, I identified myself as a healthcare worker returning from Liberia. He immediately halted his computer data entry and ordered me to follow him to another area.

I was led to a small, enclosed waiting room where a dozen other Liberians and returning healthcare workers were confined. A nurse wearing a face shield, mask, gown, and gloves, called us up one by one and our temperatures were taken. I then sat for another 20 minutes while other individuals were called for an interview with an Ebola screener.

At 3:30 p.m. my name was finally called, and I followed a masked and gloved screener to yet another enclosed area of the airport. He asked a few questions, such as my name, address, and contact information. As soon as he heard that I was in an actual Ebola Treatment Unit, he ordered me to stand and moved me to an isolation room furnished with a cot, sink, and toilet. I was soon joined by an ER physician who had briefly worked in the same Bong County ETU where I trained. He was sent home early because there were no new Ebola patients there.

We waited as screeners, public health advisors, and doctors scurried around outside our door, deciding who could be released and who required further screening or continued isolation. After thirty minutes the ER doctor sharing the isolation room with me was privately interviewed by a physician and public health advisor. In the interim, I was moved outside to a small corner space. I felt like I was in "Time Out", the notorious purgatory of bad childhood behavior. The ER physician was finally released, and I returned to the isolation room alone.

It was now 4:00 p.m., and I told the screener outside that my flight to Austin was at 5:00 p.m., and I would really like to make it. "No problem," he said.

And I waited. At 4:30 p.m. the doctor and health care advisor returned to interview me. I repeated my Liberia story once more, telling them my last Ebola contact was over 60 days ago, and I felt fine. Didn't matter. My temperature was taken once more, questions were asked, forms were filled out, and data entered into computers.

I was given a cell phone with the phone number to the Center for Disease Control Ebola hotline already programed into it. I was given another thermometer (I was up to 3 so far during my journey home). I was instructed to take my temperature twice a day. I was given forms to record my temperature along with several information sheets on the signs and symptoms of Ebola. Duh, what do you think I have been doing the past 3 months?

It was 4:45 p.m., and I told them once more that my flight would be leaving in 15 minutes. "No problem, just about done."

I was finally released and raced out of the screening area at 4:50 pm, pushing a luggage cart that held my three heavy suitcases. I threw the suitcases on the luggage conveyer belt and half ran/race walked towards my departure gate. I arrived right at 5:00 pm to find my plane still at the gate, but the doors to board were closed. I looked around for an airline employee but there were none at the desk. I heard someone on the other side of the closed door and knocked loudly, but no one came.

I saw an airline employee at a neighboring desk and ran over to see if they could assist me. I pointed to my airplane still waiting at the gate and expressed my extreme desire to be on board. "Sorry sir, once the doors are locked, no one can board."

I stood there looking out as my ride home pulled away from the gate. Forty-eight hours of sleep deprived travel and 3 months without family had broken me down emotionally and mentally. I just about cried. And so I did, but only briefly because I am a Texas kind of guy, and real Texas guys don't cry. And then it was off to the airline assistance desk to check out my travel options.

It was how I expected it to be, no other flights to Austin that night on any airline. The next flight to Austin was 8 am the next day. I was rebooked for the morning flight and given a voucher for a steeply discounted rate at a nearby

Hilton.

I walked tiredly to see if my luggage made it on the flight to Austin.

Good news. My luggage made it.

Bad news. "Welcome to Washington, D.C.!"

I walked outside to catch the shuttle bus to the Hilton. I was only wearing a long sleeve T-shirt and sweater vest that was more fashion than warmth, but it was the warmest clothes I had after living in Africa the past few months. I immediately noticed that I could see my breath and experienced a strange sensation on my skin ...it was freezing cold! Everyone around me at the shuttle stop was wearing a thick parka or a heavy black wool dress coat, this being Washington, D.C.   I could only stand outside for a few minutes before I was chilled and fled to the warmth of the terminal. I monitored the airport traffic from the sliding glass doorway and eventually saw the Hilton bus pull up. I charged through the cold to claim a spot on the bus and took the brief ride to the hotel.

The shuttle bus was filled with airline pilots and stewardesses who were happy to be getting off work. The shuttle bus station was crowded with other buses loading passengers and attempting to maneuver out of the shuttle jam. Our driver pointed the nose of our bus into the outside left lane and accelerated. Another shuttle bus to our left and slightly behind us was trying to gain access to the same lane and honked repeatedly. Our driver ignored the honking and dominated. Our shuttle driver must have taken part of his training in Liberia.

The Dulles Hilton Hotel was a magnificent, new

structure with a two story lobby, bar, and restaurant. I got a room, ordered a steak and a bottle of wine from room service, and cruised by the bar to grab a top shelf margarita to drink while my meal was prepared. I went by the hotel gift shop and picked out a hooded sweatshirt for warmth. It was turquoise blue and had Washington D.C. printed on the front in large white letters.   It screamed, "Tourist. Please rob me!"

The hotel room was beautiful with two queen beds covered by thick, luxurious, white comforters. It had a desk, lounge chair, and gleaming white-tiled bathroom. After my two- month campout in Liberia, it was downright opulent. The steak arrived, and it was the best cow meat ever. I washed it down with a bottle of Pinot Noir from California. I placed a 5 am wake-up call and collapsed into bed at 9 pm.

I woke spontaneously at 3:25 am. My warped, jet lagged brain was playing tricks on me. I tried to fall back asleep but eventually gave up and climbed out of bed to shave, shower, and start gulping down cups of coffee. I put on the same jeans and shirt that I had worn the past two days and pulled the new D.C. sweatshirt over my head. I caught the hotel shuttle to the airport, breezed through airport security, and caught my plane to Austin.

I was assigned a seat on the aisle, and there was a young woman seated next to me by the window. I made small talk with her, and eventually told her I was just returning from Liberia after working in an Ebola treatment unit. She made a forced smile. The plane had plenty of open seats, and shortly after takeoff, the young woman got up and moved across the aisle to a seat as far away from me as possible. Welcome home Ebola healthcare worker!

The flight from Washington, D.C. to Austin was a brief three hours, and we arrived ahead of schedule. My wife and brother were waiting for me at the airport, and I was looking forward to reuniting with them.

As I departed the plane and entered the terminal, I saw three official looking individuals, with nametags, examining me. They were from the Travis County Health Department and had been anticipating my arrival. They were polite and friendly, and I even received a handshake from one. One of them was a former patient of mine from many years ago when I was in private practice.

They led me to a large, enclosed office space in a secure area of the airport. We were accompanied by an airport security guard. I had my temperature taken and the list of Ebola symptoms were reviewed once more. I was shown a contract that outlined the rules for my next twenty-one days of quarantine. It stated that I would not provide any healthcare, and I would not travel by commercial or public transportation. I had to agree to stay away from large congregate settings, such as grocery stores, restaurants, churches, and theaters. I also had to take my temperature twice daily with one being visually monitored. If I failed to adhere to any of the above measures, then I would be subject to a communicable disease order.

I theorized that a communicable disease order might involve enforced confinement (Jail?) or Travis County Sheriff patrol cars parked outside my home. I went ahead and signed the contract, although I believe it was based more on public misperception and politics than science. I was just not in the mood to fight city hall.

I was given another thermometer (count now up to 4) and led out to the far end of the baggage claim area. My wife and brother were somewhere in the airport, but I didn't know where.

I walked over to the Barbara Jordan statue and texted my location. I gazed around at all the white people in a hurry to pick up their luggage and rush off to their next appointment or destination. What's the rush? Don't you know you already live in one of the richest countries in the world?

I heard my name being called, and I turned around to see my wife and brother rapidly approaching. June gave me a big hug and whispered, "Hello White Man" in my ear. I gave her a kiss on the cheek and replied, "Hello White Woman." I was home.

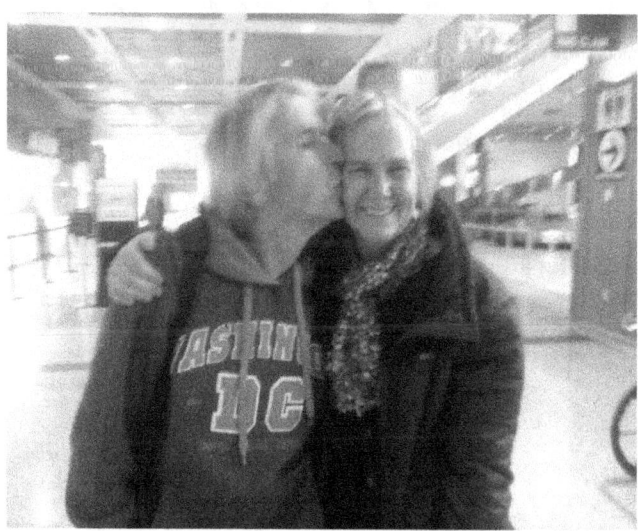

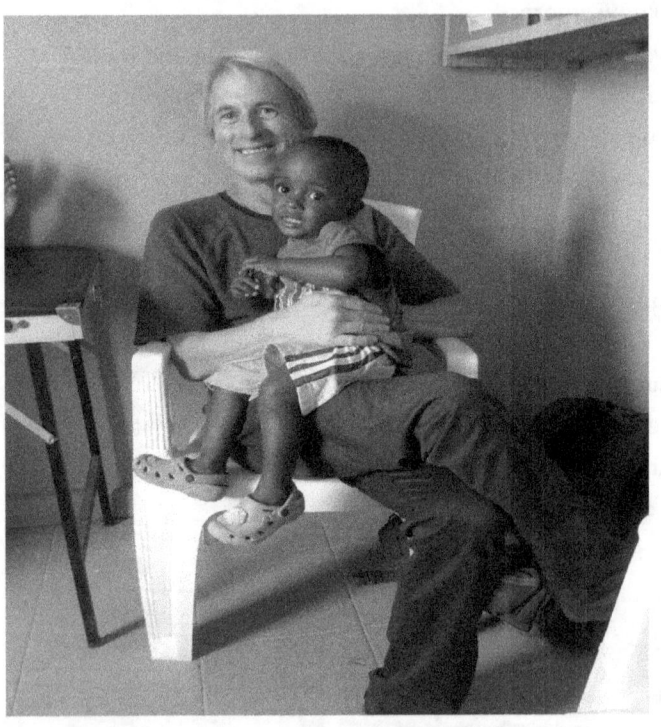

Dr. Joe Spann lives in Austin, Texas with his wife, dog, and one hundred year old cat. He continues to practice medicine at a volunteer medical clinic in Austin. This is his first book.